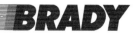

THE EMS INCIDENT MANAGEMENT SYSTEM

EMS OPERATIONS FOR MASS CASUALTY AND HIGH IMPACT INCIDENTS

Hank T. Christen, MPA, EMT
Paul M. Maniscalco, BS, EMT/P

Prentice Hall, Upper Saddle River, New Jersey 07458

Library of Congress Cataloging-in-Publication Data

Christen, Hank.
    The EMS Incident Management Systems : EMS
operations for mass casualty and high impact incidents /
by Hank Christen & Paul Maniscalco.
      p. cm.
    Includes index.
    ISBN 0-89303-972-1
    1. Disaster medicine.   2. Emergency medical services.
I. Maniscalco, Paul. II. Title.
RA645.5.C49 1998   97-53270
362.18'068—dc21   CIP

Publisher: Susan Katz
Acquisitions editor: Judy Streger
Managing development editor: Lois Berlowitz
Development editor: Arlene Bregman
Editorial/production: Elm Street Publishing Services, Inc.
Editorial/production supervision: Janet McGillicuddy
Managing production editor: Patrick Walsh
Director of production/manufacturing: Bruce Johnson
Prepress/manufacturing buyer: Ilene Sanford
Editorial assistant: Carol Sobel
Electronic page make-up: Elm Street Publishing
    Services, Inc.
Creative director: Marianne Frasco
Cover design: Joe Sengotta

©1998 by Prentice-Hall, Inc.
A Simon & Schuster Company
Upper Saddle River, New Jersey 07458

Printed in the United States of America
10 9 8 7 6 5 4 3 2

ISBN 0-89303-972-1

Notice: The author and the publisher of this
book have taken care to make certain that the
equipment and schedules of treatment are correct and compatible with the standards generally
accepted at the time of publication. Nevertheless,
as new information becomes available, changes in
treatment and in the use of equipment and procedures become necessary. The reader is advised
to carefully consult the instruction and information material included in the piece of equipment
or device before administration. First responders
are warned that the use of any techniques must
be authorized by their medical adviser, where
appropriate, in accord with local laws and regula-
tions. The publisher disclaims any liability, loss,
injury, or damage incurred as a consequence,
directly or indirectly, of the use and application
of any of the contents of this book.

Prentice-Hall International (UK) Limited, *London*
Prentice-Hall of Australia Pty. Limited, *Sydney*
Prentice-Hall Canada Inc., *Toronto*
Prentice-Hall Hispanoamericana, S. A., *Mexico*
Prentice-Hall of India Private Limited, *New Delhi*
Prentice-Hall of Japan, Inc., *Tokyo*
Simon & Schuster Asia Pte. Ltd., *Singapore*
Editora Prentice-Hall do Brasil, Ltda., *Rio de Janeiro*

BRIEF CONTENTS

CONTENTS

7   COMMUNICATIONS   75

8   THE CHEMICAL ENVIRONMENT   90

9 COMMUNITY THREAT ASSESSMENT   101

10 RESPONSE AGENCY MANAGEMENT SYSTEMS   116

11 TRAINING AND IMPLEMENTATION   132

12 EMS INCIDENT MANAGEMENT IN THE REAL WORLD   140

DEDICATION

This book is dedicated to the men and women of EMS past, present, and future. It is especially dedicated to those in Okaloosa County, Florida, and New York City, New York, who toil in the trenches daily to ensure the highest quality of pre-hospital care is available to those who require it in their time of need. It is the actions of these individuals that truly allow EMS to be defined as a profession.

FOREWORD

This book is about a really important subject. It is about how emergency service workers effectively help people who are in the wrong place at the wrong time and who get beat up and sometimes killed. The exceptional focus of the book is how to provide such services when a lot of people are in this unfortunate situation. As emergency responders, we sadly have a very limited capability to prevent such situations. Why did Mrs. Smith decide to visit her CPA in the World Trade Center on the day a group of whackos decided to drive (and detonate) a rent-a-bomb into the basement? Why did little Billy get on school bus #17 instead of #16 on the day #17 blapps into or gets blapped by some equally large vehicle? Who the hell knows?

These are unanswerable questions. The single simple question we can answer is: When such incidents happen, who does the community call? Bingo—us (right answer). At that point, the body politic needs our services badly and expects us to respond quickly, solve the problem, and be nice. Easy to say, hard to do. In fact, in most cases the customers have already paid for those services (over and over), so if we can't perform, we're really taking money under false pretenses.

Showing up when smoke is showing all over the tallest occupied building in a town with lots of really tall buildings, or arriving at an intersection with a very large upside down yellow school bus full of third graders that appears to be mated to a Westinghouse Model 342x7xhd (heavy duty) diesel locomotive with a mile and a half of freight cars behind it is, to say the least, a humongous mess. These large scale medical incidents are the most difficult situations we encounter. This book presents details of how we can move such a monstrous situation from being out of control to being under control. Again, easy to say, hard to do.

It is a blessing for the community that these big deals don't occur very often. But the infrequency of these events is also a curse for the effectiveness of our mass casualty system. There is typically a lot of time, space, and location between these Super Bowl sized medical big deals. This space creates a huge challenge for us to have the system in place and to have practiced that system when it is needed. The reality of our business is that we must use routine local, everyday small-scale events that occur all the time to set the stage of how we will operate when the infrequent "big one" hits.

The authors use the "IMS Toolbox" approach throughout the book to describe how the system expands to match the speed, size, and severity of the event. This requires system managers to continually set up and master the basic system in the beginning of every incident, so that using the system becomes instinctive and natural. We need to always be prepared to quickly and pessimistically expand the system when we encounter exceptional situations. We all must be aware that day-to-day routine medical customers that come in onesies and twosies can become a sucker punch and turn right into the middle of an "oh #!*#" situation.

While day-to-day command operations become the launching pad for big responses, we live in a dream world if we think (actually fantasize) that effective large scale medical operations will naturally and easily gallop out of what we do everyday. This text describes in detail how the management system attempts to get a lot of responders from different agencies, disciplines, and jurisdictions to play nice together. Tough to do with our naturally aggressive, independent, "Who the hell are you, son?" attitude, so pay attention to the details as you digest the material. For all you speed readers, this "ain't" a book to skim through. Effective mass casualty operations work because many details come together and work when needed. Many details work during tough conditions only because smart, hard-working, hard-headed, committed people put a "before," "during," and "after" on the system. This book describes all three stages.

As a young operations division chief (25 years ago), I sat around a table in the back of an old, decrepit inner city fire station with my able band of colleagues and, with them, developed the Phoenix Command System. A major part of that effort involved deciding, writing, and practicing and then redeciding, rewriting, and practicing some more how we would handle medical stuff. Like most places, we had (and still have) a lot of that medical stuff in Phoenix. I remember we would use poker chips to represent injured and DRT (dead right there) customers to try to somehow figure out how to build a system to take care of them. The different colored chips were different triage levels. We moved the chips around, stacked them, threw them at each other, and sometimes we'd lose some (just like in the field). If you watched us you would have thought you were looking in on a bunch of idiots playing poker with a bunch of chips and tactical worksheets instead of cards. This process went on for two or three years (literally) and created the system we have used for the past 20 years. If this book had been available then, it would have saved me enough time that I could have learned to play the piano. So, Paul and Hank, you are retrospectively the reason I am a musical klutz.

Christen and Maniscalco (responsible for my not being able to carry a note) are both interesting characters. They are basically street guys who started at the bottom, went to school, paid attention, and worked their way up through their own systems. They both have survived and prospered in large, tough, urban places where all the ammo is live and where they give you the test right before the lesson. They are both part of the "new breed" of savvy, young (to me) emergency service leaders who have inherent intelligence, practical experience, and applied education to lead us through the next wave of development within our business. They talk and write (thankfully) in plain understandable English, think in management terms, and can translate complicated stuff into doable, expandable operations with no mumbo jumbo. I have known them a long time and like them a great deal.

Like the authors, I have been a student of emergency incident command and management system development and application throughout my entire career. I have also had the opportunity to engage as a local fire officer (serving in every rank) in the ongoing development of those command and operations systems within the Phoenix Fire Department. I was here before we did IMS and I have been here after—after is better. Although, like everyone else's command system , ours is, and always will be, a work in progress. The result of all our system development is that we have created smarter command answers and organizational responses to the basic challenges that occur to us all everyday. At the end of each day, probably the most difficult and unforgiving question that continually emerges out of this development process is "are we ready?" I always stare at the ceiling and review my answers to that basic question before I go nighty-night. The place where I always think and wonder the longest is when I imagine a whole mob of seriously scuffed-up customers whose only chance of another day at the park depends on whether we can quickly deliver large-scale, effective, hard-hitting medical operations. Being able to actually apply the material in this book provides the best answers I have seen to that question. It's our job to make ourselves look like the template Christen and Maniscalco have created—let's get busy.

Alan V. Brunacini

PREFACE

Mass casualties or high-impact incidents tax any EMS agency or provider. Daily the media inform us about mass casualty incidents (MCI) occurring in every corner of America.

The causes of an MCI are multiple and varied. Natural, technological, and transportation incidents head the list. With increasing population density, the impact of these incidents will increase. New problems have emerged, such as hazardous materials and wildfire disasters in the wildland/urban interface.

Unfortunately, terrorism and criminal activity are a growth industry. We are all familiar with major incidents, such as the bombings in Oklahoma City, New York World Trade Center, and Atlanta. Daily there are smaller incidents caused by self-styled militia, street gangs, criminal enterprises, religious/political ideology groups, and disgruntled individuals. In each case, one tactical result was the creation of a high-impact event.

This book is for the responders and planners who must confront mass casualties. The authors make no distinction among response agencies. This text applies to third-service EMS, fire/EMS, private providers, volunteers, military units, EMS units in other agencies, and industrial response teams.

The subject material is applicable to all levels of the EMS organizational hierarchy. It is a text for students and teachers, a "street-wise" operations guide for responders and supervisors, and a planning guide for EMS managers, fire officers, military officers, and business contingency planners. To ensure that academic concepts reach the street, the authors have included practical implementation steps, protocols, and appendices of checklists and forms.

The boilerplate for effective mass casualty and disaster operations is the national Incident Management System (IMS). The system began as a wildfire incident command system and evolved into an urban fire command system. The EMS community has been slow to assimilate IMS. It is the intent of this book to change that. IMS provides all of us with common terminology, effective resource allocation, a functionally based system, and a system that applies to any type of risk. Since IMS is based on the military principles of command and control, civilian agencies can use the IMS to readily interface with the military and federal law enforcement agencies.

The reality of twenty-first century economics is that public and private response agencies are expected to do "more with less." Our arena is a funding/resource scarce environment. However, due to the "CNN factor," and action television/movies, public perception is one of high expectation. In other words, we're the heroes that always show up and know what to do.

MCIs and disasters present management problems as well as technical problems. These incidents must not be chaotic; disasters can and must be managed.

ACKNOWLEDGMENTS

To my wife, Lynne, and sons, Eric and Ryan, for their undying support; to Dad, District Chief (ret.) Henry T. Christen, Sr., Miami Fire Department; to Mom, Louisa Christen, who is always a giver. I'd like to thank Ms. Joyce Lee, a tireless and patient typist; Publisher Susan Katz, who saw many deadlines missed; and the many people in my life who set high standards for me to follow: David Chamberlin, Lou Cuneo, Phil Chovan, Claude Lemke, Elmer "Mac" McDonnell, Dr. Ron Weed, and Dr. David Goetsch. Special thanks to the Atlanta Fire Department and Okaloosa County Emergency Services for thirty years of adventure. Finally, thanks to co-author Paul M. Maniscalco, a friend and partner.

Hank Christen

To my wife, Connie, whose unwavering support, encouragement, and love help me to successfully achieve a balance of home and work; to my father, Anthony S. Maniscalco, who is my role model and taught me that nothing is achieved without hard work and dedication; to my mother, Patricia O'Brien Maniscalco, whose guidance over the years has taught me that kindness, compassion, and assisting others in their time of need is indeed a noble virtue; to my brothers Peter, Mark, John, and Matthew, whose support is invaluable and constant; to Susan Katz for enduring our schedules even when they were in conflict with production of this text and for continuing to support us in this endeavor; to Alan Brunacini, role model, mentor, and friend; to Jim "Spanky" Allen, MacNeil Cross, James Denney, Gerald Dickens, Walter Drivet, John Fitzsimmons, David Handschuh, Erik Gaull, Jerry Gombo, Ed Gabriel, Robert "Iceman" Iannarelli, Lynn Klein, Michael Latessa, Don Lee, Russ McCallion, Bob Morrone, Michael Newberger, Dennis Rubin, John Sinclair, Clark Staten, Mark Steffens, Robert Sudol, Julio Urbina, and Don Hiett, all of whom have been a positive influence on my professional development and career; to Matt Streger, who destroyed my theory on interns; to Jud Fuller, who believed in me, giving me a shot at EMT school at 17; lastly, to Hank Christen, my friend and co-author, who is the best!

Paul M. Maniscalco

ABOUT THE AUTHORS

Henry T. Christen, Jr., MPA, EMT, is Director of Emergency Services, Okaloosa County, Florida. He retired after sixteen years as a Battalion Chief, Atlanta Fire Department. He is the Unit Commander for the Gulf Coast Disaster Medical Assistance Team (DMAT), deploying to Hurricane Andrew (Miami) and Hurricane Marilyn. Christen served with Paul Maniscalco on the Medical Support Unit during the 1996 Atlanta Olympic bombing and is an active writer, speaker, and seminar leader. He is a consultant for private industry, local governments, and the Department of Defense in the fields of hazardous materials and incident management. Hank is a native of Miami and a graduate of the University of Florida.

Paul M. Maniscalco, BS, EMT/P, is a Deputy Chief with FDNY Bureau of EMS. His previous assignments have included Commanding Officer of the EMS Special Operations Division, EMS Emergency Manager, Manhattan North Commander and Deputy Chief of Communications. Chief Maniscalco has over twenty years of emergency response and management experience. He has published articles in numerous journals and has lectured extensively throughout North America. Maniscalco is an adjunct faculty member with the National Emergency Training Center, National Fire Academy and has worked as a consultant to many federal agencies and organizations on issues revolving around emergency incident response management and safety. Maniscalco is also a past president of the National Association of Emergency Medical Technicians.

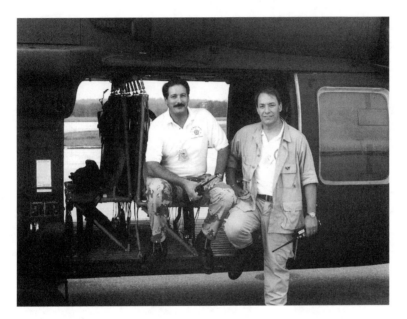

Paul M. Maniscalco (l.) and Hank Christen (r.) during medical operations at the 1996 Olympics in Atlanta.

1

THE BASICS OF INCIDENT MANAGEMENT SYSTEMS

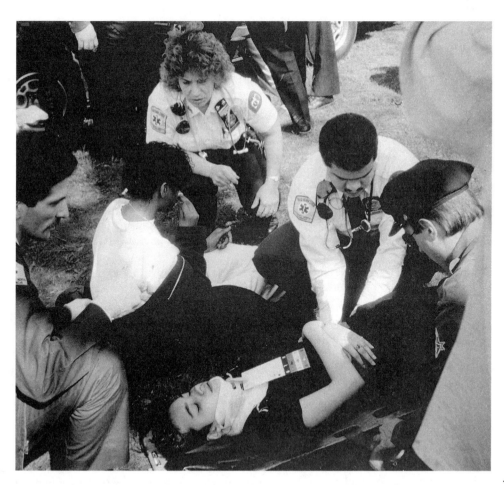

Chapter Objectives

After reading this chapter, you will be able to accomplish the following objectives:

1. Understand the history of incident management.
2. Recognize the parallels between incident management and military command structures.
3. Understand the development of fire command systems.
4. Recognize the modern management principles that are inherent in incident command systems.
5. Have a basic knowledge of the EMS Incident Management System.

THE EARLY TIMES

How far back in history do basic organizational principles go? You might guess that incident command principles were first discussed by Phoenix Fire Chief Alan Brunacini in the 1970s. Others would suggest that the writings of Peter Drucker in the 1950s and 1960s were early works on the subject. Management scholars select the writings of Henri Fayol, Chester Barnard, or Fredrick Taylor, dating back to the turn of the century. Actually, management principles were discussed several thousand years ago.

MILITARY INFLUENCES

In pre-Roman times armies were disorganized hordes. Looting and plundering were the plan of the day. The leader was the person that killed his upstarts. In a battle, the leader was always in the middle of the melee with his troops. (This still happens in many emergency medical organizations.)

The Romans changed military history. A centurion class of military professionals evolved. The famous Roman Legions were structurally organized into succinct units. The various divisions were headed by highly trained and professional leaders. Significantly, these leaders coordinated with the central commander in accordance with a plan. This form of organization continued to develop through centuries.

During the Civil War, weapons development received historical attention. The fact that improved management and control made an equal contribution to military prowess was not recognized.

In World War II several failed invasions revealed the need for developing a modern battle plan. Military leaders learned that dedicated soldiers and modern weapons were not enough. Management techniques were recognized as having equal importance with fighting skills.

These management concepts were fine tuned in Korea and Vietnam. The concepts of command, control, and communications were refined to a science in the Persian Gulf.

The management lessons learned in combat operations were also applied to the management of casualties. The first ambulances in America were wagons assigned to carry wounded soldiers in the Civil War. Patients were transported to large casualty assembly areas behind the lines.

In World Wars I and II, large field hospitals were established. For the first time, triage was developed. Patients were sorted, with the least critical receiving emergency treatment and being sent back immediately to the fighting lines. Critical patients were forwarded to surgical wards and hospital ships.

In the Korean War, the first use of helicopter patient transfer occurred. Field hospitals (MASH units) were established close to the battle front. The time from a severe wound to a surgical suite was greatly reduced. In Vietnam this time was a matter of hours. There was extensive use of helicopter transport from the immediate battle scene to sophisticated surgical units. Effective triage and advanced medical techniques led to reduced loss of life.

The lessons learned from the military operations lead us into the modern area of incident management. The lessons of war became the foundations of the first civilian incident management system.

MODERN FIRE COMMAND SYSTEMS

In the 1970s, a series of catastrophic brush fires destroyed thousands of structures. Fire units were not coordinated. There were horror stories about incompatible radio frequencies, lack of priority resource allocation, and poor coordination and control among a myriad of federal, state, and local agencies.

The lessons learned by the Roman Legions had to be relearned. The result was the California Firescope (Firefighting Resources of Southern California Organized Against Potential Emergency) Program. Key agencies began to meet and talk about mutual problems.

During the development of Firescope, emergency agencies and planners agreed on several objectives:

1. A system of command, where a single individual (or unified command team) is responsible for the ultimate outcome of the incident.
2. A system of common terminology. All agencies should understand each other.
3. A system of coordination among diversified agencies.
4. A communications system with shared frequencies and common radio language.
5. A system for resource allocation, including prioritizing and staging.

A national Incident Command System (ICS) evolved. It was determined that situations had the components of administration, planning, logistics, and operations. These sections were coordinated by an Incident Commander, supported by the Command Staff.

ICS was recognized as a system for fire agencies. Other agencies, on the outside looking in, pushed for a system that incorporated non-fire organizations into the command plan. This system was the evolutionary step that lead to the National Interagency Incident Management System (NIIMS).

ICS and NIIMS were criticized in some fire service circles as being wild-fire/California oriented. The urban fire service in the 1970s began to move in its own directions. New York City developed a command system based on operational sectors. In Phoenix, Chief Alan Brunacini developed the command system that made him famous through his excellent NFPA Fire Command Seminars. Simultaneously, David Chamberlin, former Atlanta Fire Chief, developed the incident command system taught at the Emergency Management Institute at Emmittsburg, Maryland.

Equally important components of the emergency response community other than fire service (law enforcement, Emergency Medical Services, etc.) began to rally for an incident command system that met the needs of their specific functional areas.

The functional area of Emergency Medical Service (EMS) found itself confronted with being buried in the existing ICS organizational chart as a small block labeled "medical unit." The "medical unit" is located in the service branch of the logistics section with no real delineation of the primary tasks required for successful EMS MCI operations.

The importance of a standard command system for EMS operations cannot be disputed, but what would the standard be? What should it be? Many different individuals and organizations have toiled over these questions. Most recently we have witnessed organizations such as the National Fire Academy, Emergency Management Institute, and the National Fire Service Incident Management Consortium assist with this standardization process by producing documents and educational programs to aid the local EMS provider with quickly ascending the command system learning curve.

The purpose of this text is to take the basic command principles set forth in those models and bring them to the student in a non-confusing, "real world" EMS fashion. The grasp of a theory is at times relatively easy. The application of that theory, successfully, is another story. It is our intent to share with you the specifics of the EMS Incident Management System and the successful application of the tasks from a "real world EMS" viewpoint.

MODERN MANAGEMENT PRINCIPLES

All the command systems discussed use basic management principles. These principles are the cornerstone of business management, military command systems, and emergency incident management.

Critical Factor:

Medical disasters can and must be managed. Management principles used in routine functions must be applied to the non-routine disaster.

UNITY OF COMMAND

Unity of command means someone is in control. This concept can mean that a "team" is in charge. (See Chapter 2.)

Every component, section, or unit has an individual responsible for performance. Unit members understand and recognize this authority. Managers understand their relationship to their superiors, their subordinates, and their peers.

SPAN OF CONTROL

The number of subordinates responsible to a leader is called the "span of control." An ideal span of control is three to five people but varies with the operations.

If a span of control is too narrow, the organization becomes management top heavy (lots of chiefs, too few Indians.) If the span of control is too wide, individual leaders cannot effectively manage the units or people under them. They cannot process the information overload from too many units.

CHAIN OF COMMAND

"Chain of command" is linked to unity of command and span of control and is defined as the flow of information from one command level to another.

There is an old military expression that says certain things (expletive deleted) flow downhill. We know information must flow vertically through the chain of command (uphill), as well as downward.

LINE AND STAFF (OPERATIONS AND SUPPORT)

Traditional business management models divide organizational functions into line functions and staff functions. The line function is the company's mission. Examples include making "widgets" in a manufacturing business or printing manuscripts for a publisher.

Staff functions provide support to the line functions. Staff responsibilities include areas such as finance, personnel, marketing (sales), etc. In incident management systems, the terms operations and support replace the business management terms of line and staff.

Operations, in the EMS Incident Management System, includes the triage, treatment, and transport of patients. Support functions include supplies, communications, planning, media coordination, and liaison with outside agencies.

A key concept of operations/support (or line and staff) is balance within the management system. Often operations are emphasized and support is minimized. The result is decreased operations. In summary, the right hand must complement what the left hand is doing.

> **Critical Factor:**
>
> In the EMS Incident Management System, balance between operations functions and support functions is vital.

C CUBED I (C³I)

Modern military command systems have a balanced command structure instead of a focus on operational tactics. The military jargon is command, control, communications, and intelligence. It is written C^3I, pronounced "see-cubed-eye."

This command and control system is similar to civilian public safety command systems. There is emphasis on coordination of operational functions (military tactics) with support functions.

Desert Storm was the classic example of effective military management. Throughout the conflict, commanders discussed their management successes instead of battle tactics. The media devoted as much coverage to logistics, planning, and communications as they did to the fighting. During interviews, top commanders often talked about destroying the enemy "command and control" structure rather than its weapons.

For years experts will analyze Desert Storm as a management model. The conclusion is: We won because of an effective management system. (As one Army officer said, "We had good C-cubed.")

THE CHECKLIST MENTALITY

Many incident management systems consist of checklists for every conceivable problem. Incident management control then involves following the rigid checklists.

Checklist systems tend to fail. First, if you encounter an incident that is not on the checklist, the management system falls apart. As an example, you may have a checklist for a fire, a tornado, or an airplane crash. None of these checklists is useful during a mass shooting or an earthquake.

Second, a checklist for an incident cannot be all inclusive. Disasters are full of surprises. It is impossible to think of everything. The checklist will never include surprises. (Remember: No plan survives contact with the enemy.)

Last, checklists do not address the coordination between elements in a management system. There must be assignments (based on checklist items) and inter-relations between the people receiving the assignments. Management systems address these relationships; checklist systems do not.

Checklists have their place. Detailed and repetitive procedures are well-suited to checklists. Inspecting a hand-held radio or setting up an oxygen cascade system requires a checklist. Equipment needs are a resource checklist. Just remember, checklists are not management systems.

MANAGEMENT FOCUS VERSUS TASK FOCUS

Tasks require the manual skills necessary to carry out an operational plan. Most tasks are hands-on operations. This includes skills such as CPR, IV therapy, bandaging, or splinting. Obviously, tasks are the essence of incident operations. When tasks are applied without management (command/control), there is no effective system. More importantly, there is no coordination and individuals (or units) operate in a freelance style. Their task skills may be excellent, but are applied at the wrong place or the wrong time.

Consider a mass casualty incident with task focus only. All the medics are treating patients and no single person is in charge. The order of treatment is "first come, first served." (The management concept of triage is missing). There are no support functions since everyone is concentrating on individual tasks. As the incident progresses, there is a depletion of EMS supplies, a breakdown in communications, and a loss of transportation resources, with no one responsible.

Whereas on a daily basis we applaud independent actions, at the scene of the MCI there is no room for independent actions. Independent actions, in these instances, lead to "freelancing," and often the actions of "freelancers" yield results that are contrary to the commanders' strategies or cause safety problems. It is evident that many EMS providers do not recognize the need for senior supervision, yet the orientation of all members of an EMS system to the behavioral requirements of the Incident Management System is a must.

The required transition is one from relationship behavior to task behavior. Usually an EMS provider has the luxury at most emergency and non-emergency calls to discuss and reason with his or her partners regarding actions to take, treatment protocols to follow, and hospitals to which to transport. This participatory decision-making process can be termed an example of relationship behavior. When an EMS crew is operating at an MCI, its actions are being dictated by a Sector Officer and crew members might find themselves being transferred from one sector to another based upon the requirements of the incident. The directions given by the Sector Officer must be followed to ensure that the overall tactics and strategies are applied as intended by the Incident Manager or Branch Director. These actions are examples of task behavior.

When a crew is operating in the MCI arena, there is no time for relationship behavior. The directions of the Sector Officer must be followed in order to ensure the efficacy of the operation and safety of all involved.

THE IMS MODEL

The national Incident Management System (IMS) is a management model that incorporates all the sound management principles discussed earlier in this chapter.

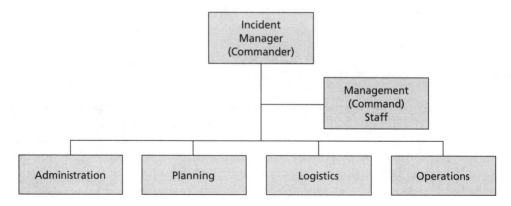

Figure 1-1 Basic Structure of the Incident Management System

The individual in charge is called the Incident Manager. The Incident Manager is assisted by a Management Staff, a group of specialists coordinating as a Manager's support team.

There are four major sections under the Management Staff. These sections are Administration, Planning, Logistics, and Operations. (See Figure 1-1.) In many cases, Administration does not justify full section status. In these situations, Administration can become a unit in another section.

This model is the basis for all public safety management systems. The system, as diagrammed, incorporates all of the elements previously discussed.

- Unified Command—There is a single person (or management team) in charge.
- Span of Control—No individual manages more than three to five sections or units.
- Chain of Command—There is a clear flow of information up or down. (Remember: Sometimes the "expletive deleted" has to flow uphill.)
- Line and Staff—There is a line function (operations), supported and coordinated with staff functions (logistics, planning, and administration).
- C^{3}I—There is a system of command, control, communications, and intelligence. (We call intelligence reconnaissance, recon, or threat assessment, in the public safety world.)
- Flexibility—The system applies to any incident (or management problem). It is not a system of checklists.

This model is generic and not specific to medical disasters. In the next section, we will develop the incident management model into the EMS Incident Management System.

INCIDENT CLASSIFICATIONS

A medical incident (non-routine) is classified as either a routine event or a mass casualty incident, also known as a multiple-casualty incident (MCI).

An MCI is an event that

- Produces several patients.
- Produces a minimal number of casualties but has unusual events surrounding the incident (e.g., Haz Mat, multiple vehicle accident, rail, aircraft, or marine incident, etc.).
- Affects local hospital(s) receiving the patients to the point that normal EMS operations become hindered, thereby having a negative impact on system efficacy.
- Generally may "draw down" the system resources, or the number of patients outnumbers the resources of initial rescuers.

A disaster is a type of MCI that involves hundreds or thousands of patients. It strikes anytime, anywhere. It takes many forms—a hurricane, an earthquake, a tornado, a flood, a fire or a hazardous spill, an act of nature or an act of terrorism. It builds over days or weeks, or hits suddenly, without warning. Every year millions of Americans face disasters and their terrifying consequences. The medical and public safety infrastructure may suffer considerable damage. Resources will be needed from the state and federal government. Operations will be conducted in what the military calls a "resource scarce environment." In a disaster, a complete EMS Incident Management System will be needed to provide planning, administration, and logistical support to operation teams.

The term MCI should be transmitted via the designated communications system. If the meaning of this term is clearly understood, other units can respond accordingly. They can activate the appropriate checklists in communications centers and medical control. All responding agencies must know the meaning of an MCI and should identify an incident as such.

A medical disaster is not declared by a responding unit. A disaster declaration unfolds after a period of damage assessment or after several days of emergency operations. In many states a governor's official declaration of emergency is required to obtain state and federal resources.

EMS Incident Management builds from the bottom level upwards. As operation units survey their situation, they build the incident management system. It begins from a single patient incident to an MCI and finally to a medical disaster, which is really an expanded MCI (Figures 1-2, 1-3, and 1-4).

EMS INCIDENT MANAGEMENT SYSTEM

The principles and organizational structure in the Fire Incident Command System are easily adopted into a EMS Incident Management System (EMS/IMS). The key components are triage, treatment, and transportation. Staging is an additional sector in a medical disaster. These tactical activities are coordinated by an EMS Branch.

The Incident Manager is supported by a Command Staff consisting of a liaison, as well as safety, public information, and trauma intervention program (TIPs) personnel. All of these sectors, and the sectors described below, may require expansion depending on the situation.

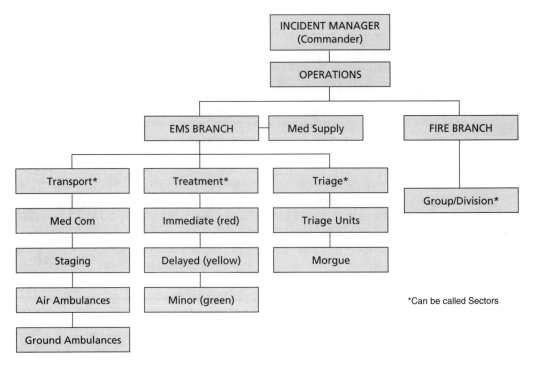

Figure 1-2 Mass Casualty Incident

The Planning Section provides documentation (medical records), planning, and administration. Rarely is an incident large enough to justify separate Administration and Planning Sections.

The Logistics Section provides support in the form of communications, medical supplies, facilities, and mobilization.

The Operations system in Figure 1-3 applies to major incidents. All diagrammed functions are not necessary in small-scale situations.

In a routine automobile accident with two patients, a single paramedic team can perform the required functions. The senior member is in charge. The team triages the patients, selects the proper supplies, applies treatment, communicates, and transports the patients.

In a larger incident, management systems must begin to function. Consider a bus accident with 15 patients.

A supervisor must assume command. The supervisor should not be touching patients. One team must concentrate on triage, since patient treatment must be prioritized. Normal transport resources will become overwhelmed. Transportation coordination becomes a function assigned to a transportation unit. Additional supplies are sent by transporting a disaster cache to the scene. One medic is assigned responsibility for EMS Supply.

A Public Information Officer (PIO) reports to the scene to coordinate media relations. A trauma intervention team is activated to conduct a post incident stress debriefing session.

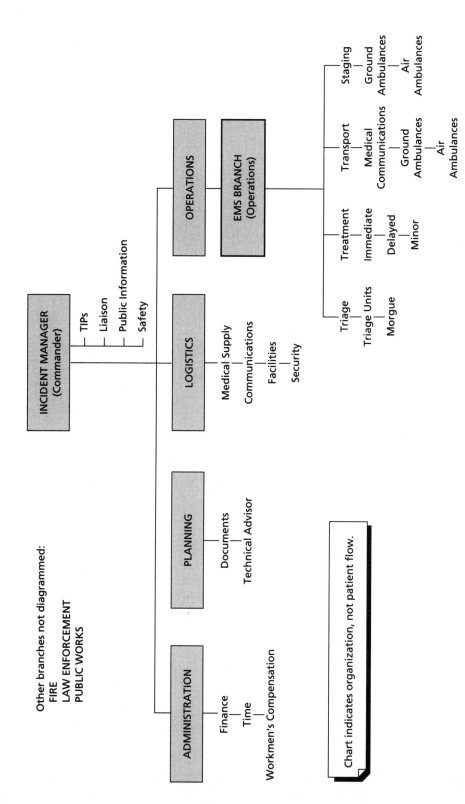

Figure 1-3 Expanded Mass Casualty Incident—An Incident Major in Scope and/or Duration

11

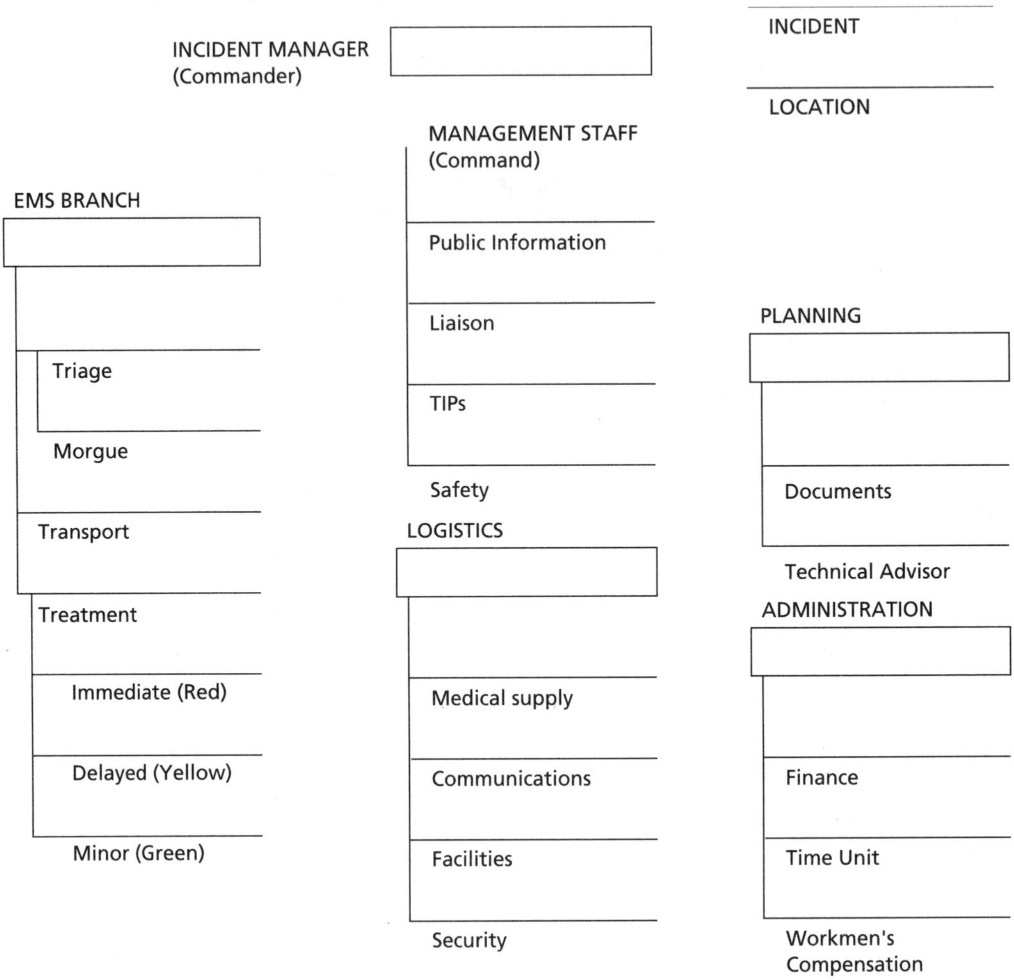

INCIDENT MANAGER
(Commander)

INCIDENT

LOCATION

MANAGEMENT STAFF
(Command)

EMS BRANCH

Public Information

Liaison

PLANNING

Triage

TIPs

Morgue

Documents

Safety

Transport

LOGISTICS

Technical Advisor

ADMINISTRATION

Treatment

Immediate (Red)

Medical supply

Delayed (Yellow)

Communications

Finance

Minor (Green)

Facilities

Time Unit

Security

Workmen's
Compensation

Figure 1-4 EMS Incident Management System

    In this incident the local EMS delivery system is stressed. Management functions (according to IMS) are assigned as needed. There is a system of control and coordination.

    Finally, suppose a medical disaster natural event has devastated an area. There are several hundred casualties. A disaster team from the region or from out-of-state must respond.

    It is necessary to fully implement IMS. The Incident Manager must deal with a large-scale and long-term operation. A full Command Staff will be necessary in addition to the PIO and TIPs. A Liaison Officer will be needed to integrate outside agencies, and a Safety Officer will be needed to coordinate safety operations.

    A Planning Section will also be needed. An Incident Action Plan must be developed and coordinated with the Incident Manager in long-term operations. A resources unit will be needed to track ambulances (both air and ground), personnel, and outside agency resources. A medical records (documentation) unit will be needed to keep patient treatment records and records of patient destinations.

A Logistics Section will provide medical supplies, communications, and facilities (including food and water) for the disaster team.

The Operations Section will have to be expanded into an EMS Branch consisting of multiple treatment areas, if the scene dictates. Triage will become a sector function. Transport will become a major sector, coordinating arrival of incoming patients and dispersal of outgoing patients. Staging will be expanded to sector level.

Each section of the EMS Incident Management System is discussed in detail in future chapters and each position in the system is described in Appendix 1.

WHERE DO THE MANAGERS COME FROM?

So far the EMS Incident Management System looks great on paper. However, the obvious question is, "Where do all of the managers come from?"

Many EMS systems do not have several tiers of mid-level managers or supervisors. In numerous cases, EMS will be working within the Fire Incident Command System. This means the Command Staff and several of the support staff may be fire service personnel. In the school bus accident previously described, some EMS systems would not have the supervisory personnel to staff the required functions. This is why the EMS Management System must be "street smart" instead of being a mere paper plan. Several important concepts must be understood.

- The elements of IMS are functions, not necessarily management positions.
- The Incident Manager assumes all functions not formally delegated. This is the foundation of the system.
- Not all IMS functions are necessary. Only the largest medical disaster requires full implementation.
- Individuals can perform more than one function.
- Section Chiefs and unit leaders do not have to come from the ranks of managers or supervisors. Any qualified person, regardless of rank, can fill a functional position in IMS.
- The system builds from the bottom up. The structure grows as the incident grows.
- The IMS is like a toolbox. You select the tools you need but rarely empty the box.

SUMMARY

The basic management concepts inherent in the EMS Incident Management System date back thousands of years. Military and business management systems are based on unity of command, chain of command, and span of control.

The modern Public Safety Incident Command System evolved from experiences in the urban fire service and from lessons learned during severe wildfire incidents in California (the California Firescope Program). These systems contained operations (line functions) and support functions (staff) and were further refined by the National Fire Service Incident Management Consortium and the National Fire Academy.

The EMS Incident Management System (IMS) is designed to respond to EMS incidents that vary from routine to medical disasters. The IMS concept utilizes a Command Staff, an Operations Section, a Logistics Section, and a Planning Section. Operations include triage, treatment, and transport (and staging in disasters). Logistics includes communications, EMS supplies, facilities, and mobilization. Planning includes an Incident Action Plan, resources status, patient records, and administration.

A mass casualty incident (MCI) has more patients than providers. Patients are triaged and treated with BLS procedures. Rapid transport of critical patients is the goal. A Medical Disaster is an expanded MCI usually caused by a natural event, technical failure, or terrorism. EMS resources are overwhelmed. Regional, state, and federal assistance are needed. The incident is long in duration.

CHAPTER QUESTIONS/EXERCISES

1. What were the main management objectives in the development of the California Firescope Program?
2. Diagram the EMS Incident Management System. Include the functions in the Command Staff, as well as the functions in the Operational and Support Sections.
3. Define the key management functions that would be necessary in the following incidents.
   a. A vehicle roll-over on an expressway during rush hour. Three vehicles are involved, two patients are critical, four patients are serious, two patients have minor injuries.
   b. A major airplane crash, two miles short of the runway in a residential area. There are 52 fatalities, 28 critical, 15 serious, and 10 minor injuries. Your agency has only eight available transport units.
   c. A tornado has struck a major urban area. There are over 200 destroyed structures. Initial reports indicate 75 fatalities and over 200 injuries of varying degree. The only trauma center in the region has been destroyed.
4. Your EMS agency does not have the supervisors or personnel to fully staff the required IMS positions. What people and/or agencies in your community could be utilized to staff the following functional positions:
   a. Logistics
   b. Trauma Intervention Program (TIPs)
   c. Public Information Officer (PIO)
   d. Resources
   e. Safety
   f. Facilities
   g. Communications

5. Examine the management system and operating procedures currently being used by your organization. Also study the area disaster plans. What key elements in Incident Management are present in these plans? What key elements in IMS are not indicated in your present incident management structure?

2

WHO'S IN CHARGE?

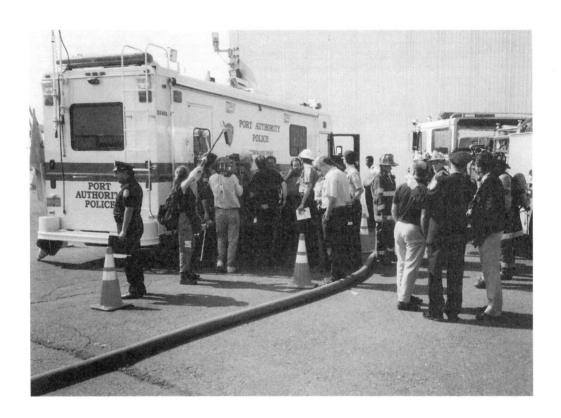

Chapter Objectives
After reading this chapter, you will be able to accomplish the following objectives:

1. Have an awareness of the duties and responsibilities of an Incident Manager.
2. Recognize the political problems and turf problems associated with leadership in an Incident Management System.
3. Understand the relationship between the EMS Branch and the Fire Incident Manager.
4. Understand the concept of Unified Management.

In some incidents, no one is in charge. In others, the wrong person is in charge. In some cases, too many people are in charge. We've all been there.

- No one is in charge—Most of us like that mode. We can operate freely without anyone bothering us. However, in a mass casualty incident (MCI), there are too many things to track. We need someone to run the show.
- The wrong person is in charge—Can you remember the last time you took orders from an Incident Manager with no EMS training? Many of us have experienced police officers running the scene. There's the horror story of EMS administrators, with no street experience, arriving to "help." The right person must be in charge.
- Too many people are in charge—The Fire Chief is in charge, the EMS Commander is in charge, and the Sheriff is in charge, simultaneously. Orders and instructions are coming from all directions. When one commander devises a plan, another commander changes it. One person, or a unified team, must be in charge.

WHAT DETERMINES WHO'S IN CHARGE?

In a single agency, it's clear who runs the organization. All organizations/agencies have "Heads of State" that preside over a precise organizational chart. Everyone knows who is the "boss."

When mass casualty incidents occur, many agencies become involved. Suddenly it is not obvious who is in command. This is true when several agency heads arrive, each expecting to manage the incident.

Command authority, when several agencies are involved, is usually determined by state legislation. The legislation specifies who should be in command. In some states, the fire chief of the appropriate jurisdiction is in charge at non-law enforcement emergencies. This includes mass casualty incidents. The approach is logical since fire departments usually have extensive emergency experience, along with communications and organizational command experience.

Most states specify that the ranking EMS professional on the scene is in charge of patient care. He/she determines the order of treatment, the type of treatment, and priority and destination of transport.

Statutes give authority to law enforcement officers to control crime scenes. State law enforcement (Highway Patrol) has operational authority on state highways. In a few states, the Highway Patrol has authority over hazardous materials incidents.

Statutes give the sheriff (an elected official) authority over all law enforcement incidents in a county. These laws give a sheriff jurisdiction over incidents that effect the general welfare of the county or its citizens. Most state legislatures give sheriffs far-reaching powers. Federal statutes, e.g., Nunn-Luger legislation, give command authority to the FBI if an incident is caused by terrorism.

Determining the Incident Manager by legislation raises many questions.

1. What about the inexperienced or poorly trained manager? Levels of sophistication vary greatly. Many agencies have no Incident Management System.
2. What happens when non-medical managers try to dictate patient treatment?
3. What happens when there are conflicts of authority? You can have a hazardous materials incident on a state highway with fire/rescue problems and injured patients.

RESOLVING TURF PROBLEMS

You want to give your patients the best medical care possible. But you're constantly at incident scenes that are defined by non-EMS individuals as "their turf." We want the public to think all agencies work together on a scene holding hands and singing "Kumbaya." This is not always the case. If you've been a street EMT or paramedic for more than a week, you've already been an unwilling participant in an inter-agency conflict.

Legislation is not a total solution. However, state and local statutes are a good place to start. Examine the laws that apply to your jurisdiction and determine who is in charge under various scenarios. Next comes the hard part. Identify the players and bring them together for consensus. This process cannot be initiated at the EMT/paramedic level. EMS management must be the facilitator.

The first goal of the committee is to develop a formal Community Disaster Plan. This plan should apply to routine incidents, mass casualty incidents, and disasters. The plan must identify who is in charge.

The Committee should answer the following questions:

1. How do EMS agencies relate to the Fire Incident Command System?
2. How is command shared with law enforcement when there are multiple victims at a crime scene?
3. When does the EMS Commander become the Incident Manager or a member of a Unified Management Team?
4. Who has management authority at transportation accidents?
5. Who is in charge at hazardous materials scenes?
6. What is the formal process for changing management during an incident? (Note: All management changes must be communicated to personnel at an incident scene.)

The answers to these questions depend on state statutes, local procedures, the Fire Incident Management System, historical precedents, and personalities. The answers comprise a formal document called the Community Disaster Plan, signed by all agency managers outlined in the Plan.

The Committee's job is never finished. There should be a review of major incidents and situations where questions of command authority have arisen. Revisions to the agency or Community Disaster Plan should be added as needed. These changes most times will become recognizable due to the results yielded from your Post Incident Analysis (PIA). Changes implemented can range from communication protocols to who has the jurisdiction for supply acquisition for logistics. In any event the inclusion of an objective process which evaluates agency performance and community risk analysis must be a vital component of the planning process.

Critical Factor:

The Incident Manager must be identified and specified in a formal Community Disaster Plan.

QUALITIES OF AN INCIDENT MANAGER

An Incident Manager should be qualified. Defining Incident Managers in a Community Disaster Plan does not mean they can do the job.

Texts in the management and public safety fields have identified the characteristics of a good manager. Based on these writings, we can define the ideal manager as:

1. All-knowing.
2. Forceful, yet sensitive.
3. Omnipotent (not impotent).
4. Totally calm under fire.
5. Likes dogs and small children.
6. Free of impure thoughts.
7. Brave, honest, clean, trustworthy.

No one can meet the requirements of this "tongue in cheek" list. But it is important that your leader have the following attributes:

1. In-depth Incident Management training. This especially applies to administrators who do not have the command experiences.
2. A thorough knowledge of the EMS Incident Management System.
3. Be familiar with the Community Disaster Plan and participate in disaster exercises.
4. Stay at a command post and not perform hands-on operations. An Incident Manager's tools are a hand-held radio and a clipboard, not a gun, fire-hose, or bandage scissors.

NOTE: The term "Incident Manager" is gender neutral.

DUTIES OF AN INCIDENT MANAGER

The Incident Manager (IM) does not "command" in the true sense of the word. The IM coordinates the major functions of operations, logistics, and planning. The IM ensures there is a flow of information, personnel, and resources between support functions and operational functions.

The word "commander" is nationally accepted terminology. However, the duties of this position are to lead and manage. Therefore, the term Incident Manager is used in this text.

As an incident increases in size, more diverse agencies play a role. This is why a military style command structure does not work. Agencies do not have to obey the Incident Manager. Therefore, the IM must depend on consensus and coordination rather then coercion (charisma and a sense of humor also help). The agencies and the IM must operate within an agreed upon management system (another plug for EMS/IMS).

The IM is responsible for the outcome of a mass casualty incident. The IM is also a liaison between the outside world and the incident scene. Resources come from outside the system and are inserted into the arena in a planned and effective manner.

The primary duties of the IM are:

1. Establish a command post.
2. Maintain a reasonable span of control by delegating major functions.
3. Delegate responsibilities for the functions of planning, logistics, and operations.
4. Assume responsibility for any functions not delegated.
5. Provide a liaison with outside agencies.
6. Provide for personnel safety (mental and physical).
7. Prioritize the allocation of scarce resources.
8. Receive and disseminate vital information among all sections of the IMS.
9. Ensure effective communications among all system elements.
10. Coordinate the development and implementation of an operational plan.
11. Coordinate accurate release of information to media agencies.
12. Terminate incident operations.
13. Produce a post incident report and critique.
14. Cooperate with post incident investigations.

The list is extensive. No individual can accomplish all these duties. The IM needs help. But the IM must assume final responsibility for the outcome of a mass casualty incident. Harry Truman's favorite expression, "The buck stops here," certainly applies to the IM. (See Figure 2-1.)

POLITICAL REALITIES

Mass casualty incidents can have political implications. First, every incident is on someone's political turf. Second, most of the people involved, including EMS professionals, are government employees. Third, the cause or outcome of an incident can have far-reaching political effects.

The IM has a political challenge. Elected officials will respond to high profile emergency scenes. Political officials may take command or make operational decisions. (This is every Incident Manager's nightmare).

Figure 2-1

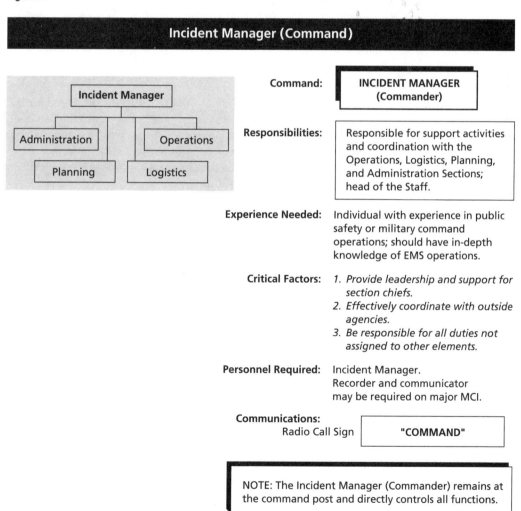

Incident Manager (Command)

Incident Manager
Administration
Operations
Planning
Logistics

Command: INCIDENT MANAGER (Commander)

Responsibilities: Responsible for support activities and coordination with the Operations, Logistics, Planning, and Administration Sections; head of the Staff.

Experience Needed: Individual with experience in public safety or military command operations; should have in-depth knowledge of EMS operations.

Critical Factors:
1. *Provide leadership and support for section chiefs.*
2. *Effectively coordinate with outside agencies.*
3. *Be responsible for all duties not assigned to other elements.*

Personnel Required: Incident Manager. Recorder and communicator may be required on major MCI.

Communications:
Radio Call Sign — **"COMMAND"**

NOTE: The Incident Manager (Commander) remains at the command post and directly controls all functions.

When political officials arrive, direct them to the command post. The IM should give the officials a short and concise briefing. Attempt to link the officials with the Public Information Officer (PIO).

The PIO must get the officials away from the operational scene and into a pristine press briefing area. Since most elected officials are interested in media exposure, this is usually acceptable. This allows officials to make a positive contribution. Because of public recognition and confidence, they are effective in informing and calming the public. That's why it is important for officials to receive updated facts and information about the situation.

If you are in an operational capacity and receive orders from elected officials, notify your supervisor immediately. This information should flow up to the IM. (This process should be done in seconds.) The IM can arrange the proper escorts. Political officials are dedicated. When they respond to a major scene, they have a concern and desire to help. Place them in the media relations mode and out of the operations mode. This can ensure a positive contribution.

UNIFIED MANAGEMENT

In the beginning pages of this chapter, we examined the responsibilities of an IM. The demands of such a long list of responsibilities can be insurmountable. In complex incidents, there are several operational objectives. A team may have to manage the incident. This form of incident management is known as Unified Management.

A Unified Management Team is needed in any scenario where operations are shared by two or more diverse organizations.

Consider the following examples:

1. A mass shooting incident where the suspect is still on the scene—operations are shared by law enforcement and Emergency Medical Services—the Unified Management Team would be police and EMS.
2. A building collapse with trapped victims and mass casualties—operations are shared by EMS and fire/rescue—the Unified Management Team would be fire and EMS.
3. A terrorist incident involving the release of a chemical agent with casualties and a large area evacuation—operations are shared by law enforcement, fire/Haz Mat, and EMS—the Unified Management Team would be police, fire, and EMS.

The Unified Management Team avoids operational confusion. Major operational areas are managed by people familiar with these functions.

On paper, the concept of Unified Management looks sound. It works when the following requirements are met:

1. The managers must coordinate and share the management turf.
2. The managers must be adequately trained in Incident Management.
3. The troops at the street level must understand how to work under Unified Management.
4. There cannot be major personality conflicts between the players on the Unified Management Team.

A Unified Management Team may be needed when a large-scale incident occurs in more than one political jurisdiction. This may happen when a city, county, or state boundary bisects the emergency scene. In these cases, managers from both jurisdictions may share management functions.

Critical Factor:

Incidents with more than one operational function, or incidents involving multiple jurisdictions, need a Unified Management Team.

SUMMARY

In emergency management systems, it is important to determine who will take charge. This can be decided by legislation, but ultimately must achieve a consensus of the agencies involved.

Major emergency incidents become political incidents. Elected officials may respond to a mass casualty scene. They should be assigned to the Public Information Officer and kept away from scene operations.

An Incident Manager is directly responsible for coordinating support functions (logistics and planning) with operational functions. The Incident Manager is responsible for liaison with the outside world.

More than one individual may be responsible for incident management. This is called Unified Management and occurs when operational functions are shared, or an incident is in more than one jurisdiction.

CHAPTER QUESTIONS/EXERCISES

1. What statutes in your state determine who is in charge of disaster incidents? What authority is given for patient care responsibility? What are the powers of sheriffs in your state?
2. What disaster plans are in effect in your community? Who is specified as the Incident Manager in the Community Disaster Plan?
3. You are the Incident Manager. A city councilman and county commissioner have entered the operational area. How would you handle this matter? How would you solve this problem if you were an EMT or paramedic on this incident?
4. List the fire chiefs in your area. What is the Incident Management training/experience background for these individuals?
5. List and define at least five duties of an Incident Manager.
6. During a recent MCI in your area, the fire chief was the Incident Manager. The chief was non-medical, but made several decisions that directly affected patient care. When confronted, the chief vehemently defended his sole authority as Incident Manager. How would you solve this problem?
7. Discuss and define the concept of Unified Management. List three scenarios where a Unified Management Team would be effective.

3

THE MANAGEMENT STAFF

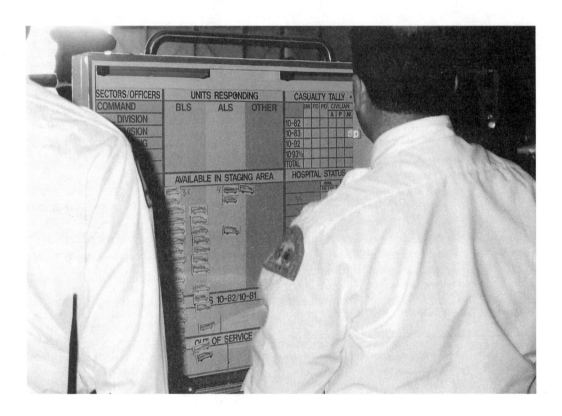

Chapter Objectives

After reading this chapter, you will be able to accomplish the following objectives:

1. Understand the concept of a Management Staff.
2. Diagram the organizational structure of the Management Staff.
3. Understand the relationship between the Incident Manager and members of the Management Staff.
4. Define the duties of the Public Information Officer, Safety Officer, Liaison Officer, and the Trauma Intervention Program (TIPs).

THE MANAGEMENT STAFF CONCEPT

In Chapter 2 we reached the conclusion that the Incident Manager has a long and demanding list of responsibilities. In a major incident, an Incident Manager cannot perform the required duties without help. This assistance comes from a Management Staff.

The Management Staff concept has proven its effectiveness in business and military management. A manager (or senior officer) has an appointed staff of specialists to provide expertise directly to him or her. You commonly hear about administrative assistants in business or staff officers in the military. In politics, there is continuous reference to congressional staffers or to the White House Staff.

In emergency incident management, the Management Staff handles the functions of safety, liaison, public information, and traumatic stress management. (See Figure 3-1.) The staff has a direct relationship with the Incident Manager. It is the Management Staff's job to assist the Incident Manager. The Management Staff is unique because it does not directly supervise major command functions (logistics, planning, operations). Staffers do not usually have subordinates, but incident size or complexity may require them.

Most of the staff positions are not physically anchored to the command post. These people move throughout the incident area depending on their duties.

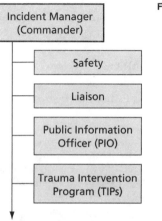

Figure 3-1 The Management Staff

They may be working in any of the functional sections or coordinating with outside agencies.

WHEN DO YOU APPOINT A STAFF?

Where does the Management Staff come from? This is a valid question since most organizations are understaffed. In an MCI, treatment personnel are overwhelmed. All available people are needed to treat patients. Therefore, a Management Staff may be perceived as a luxury rather than a necessity.

Two critical points serve as guidelines when appointing a Management Staff:

First, remember the cornerstone of Incident Management. Any duties not assigned by the Incident Manager are assumed to be the Incident Manager's responsibility. In minor incidents, the Incident Manager can monitor safety, serve as a liaison to the other agencies, and give brief media statements. As complications arise, or as the incident increases in size, these responsibilities become too demanding and the Incident Manager must assign staff to necessary functions.

Second, Management Staff positions do not require medical professionals when confronted with large-scale or high-impact events. Paramedics and EMTs are needed in the Operations Section for these instances. The liaison, safety, public information, and stress management personnel *can* be professionals in other fields. The Safety Officer can be a fire officer or safety inspector. The Liaison Officer can be a fire officer, Emergency Management director, or EMS administrator. The Public Information Officer should be the jurisdiction's public affairs professional. Stress debriefing should be conducted by a local or regional team.

> **Critical Factor:**
>
> The Management Staff should be assigned as needed. Staff functions should be performed by trained specialists, not emergency medical professionals.

MANAGEMENT STAFF SCENARIOS

The following scenarios demonstrate effective use of Management Staffs:

1. Automobile accident with five victims and two fatalities—The Incident Manager serves as a liaison with law enforcement. The Incident Manager monitors safety and is able to give a statement to a media crew. There is no need for stress debriefing on the scene. In this scenario there is no Management Staff. Instead, the Incident Manager has assumed all staff functions.

2. School bus rollover with 10 minor injuries, 8 critical injuries, and 4 fatalities—The Incident Manager performs liaison duties with outside agencies. Since extensive

extrication is involved, a fire training officer is selected as a Safety Officer. The city's public relations specialist serves as the PIO. The Incident Manager calls the trauma intervention program to deal with the victim's parents. In this scenario the Management Staff consists of safety, public information, and stress management personnel.

3. Major airline crash in a residential area with 75 fatalities and 50 injuries—From the onset, the Incident Manager realizes this is a mass casualty incident and a full Management Staff will be needed. The Incident Manager assigns a Battalion Chief to coordinate safety functions. The Director of Emergency Management is assigned as the Liaison Officer. The county Public Affairs Officer arrives and establishes a media team with airline and government PIOs. The Trauma Intervention Unit is immediately called. It will assist on the scene and schedule a stress defusing session for the next duty day. Throughout this incident, the Management Staff coordinates with the Incident Manager.

The preceding scenarios provide a varied range of incidents. In the one case in which there is no Management Staff, the Incident Manager assumes the duties. At the other end of the spectrum, there is a full Management Staff that may operate for several days and incorporate multiple agencies or functional areas. When you need a staff, assign the appropriate people. If you don't need a staff, don't waste your most valuable resource—personnel.

THE STRESS MANAGEMENT CONCEPT

In public safety circles, trauma intervention programs for both acute and long-term treatment of traumatic stress is still a relatively new concept. The emotional toll that emergency services can have on members was not appreciated nor understood until just recently.

The "macho code" governed a predominantly male organization. Emergency services professionals were perceived as emotionally tough. People were not supposed to be psychologically affected by their work: "Real men and women didn't cry."

We now recognize that emotional reactions to the stresses of our job is quite human. Emergency incidents involve an enormous potential for producing high emotional stress. We see human suffering that can include hideous trauma or dismemberment. We confront the death of children. Unfortunately, we sometimes see serious injury or death of fellow workers.

The concept of trauma intervention is that emotional maintenance is as important as equipment maintenance. We acknowledge equipment has to be inspected, maintained, and repaired, but we dismiss thoughts that people won't operate at 100% capability. The uninformed Incident Manager believes that the members "will deal with it." But this is just not the case. Acute or cumulative events can and do affect members. Therefore, utilization of the trauma intervention process helps to maintain our people.

Trauma Intervention Teams are formal organizations with a Director (usually a mental health professional). Team members have a formal training process.

Peer support is essential since many emergency workers trust their colleagues but may not trust doctors, psychologists, etc. Trauma intervention experts caution the use of mental health professionals not familiar with emergency services, not trained or suited for disaster operations.

The job of the Trauma Intervention Team begins before the incident. An effective team will conduct training for all emergency services personnel. This acquaints emergency professionals with the team members and exposes people to the Trauma Intervention Program philosophy. It also teaches stress reducing techniques. Most of all, it demonstrates that emotional reaction is normal and help is available.

During the incident, the Trauma Intervention Team provides on-scene support. The Trauma Intervention Officer advises the Incident Manager about stress-related matters. Reduction of noise, effective scene control, and assisting in the emotional care of victims' families can diminish the stressful atmosphere of an emergency. Other techniques include rest and rotation periods for workers and pre-deployment briefings for arriving personnel. (See Figure 3-2.)

Immediately after the incident, the Trauma Intervention Team conducts a defusing session. This is followed by a debriefing session within 24 to 72 hours. In some cases, individuals may require longer-term counseling with licensed mental health professionals.

An Incident Manager should remember:

1. People are the most important asset in emergency services.
2. A Trauma Intervention Team should be part of the management system.
3. If you think a Trauma Intervention Team may be needed, you should have already called them.

SAFETY

Physical safety of emergency personnel is as important as emotional safety. Disasters are dangerous places to work and operate. The area can be on fire or have hazardous chemicals present. There may be partially collapsed structures, downed wires, and debris. Severe weather and darkness can be threatening. Power tools, equipment, and vehicles are being operated. In terrorist and law enforcement incidents, there may be explosive devices or people with weapons (good guys and bad guys). Disasters are bad places to work.

Another danger factor is the mindset of medical professionals and emergency workers. We are action-oriented people. We recognize positive action. We want to arrive at an incident and control it. We take chances without considering safety, never recognizing ourselves as potential victims.

The Incident Manager is responsible for the safety of everyone on the scene. Considering the conditions at a disaster, coupled with the mindset of the

Figure 3-2

Trauma Intervention Program

Staff:	TRAUMA INTERVENTION PROGRAM
Responsibilities:	Trauma Intervention Program (TIPs); interacts with all members to help reduce and defuse emotional stress; conducts post-incident stress debriefings.
Experience Needed:	Individual with formal TIPs training and working knowledge of EMS operations.
Critical Factors:	1. *Provide emotional support to personnel working under conditions of extreme physical and emotional stress.* 2. *Coordinate with Command in eliminating stress conditions.*
Personnel Required:	TIPs Team members.
Communications: Radio Call Sign	**"TIPs"**

Staff support for Incident Manager (Commander).

NOTE: The TIPs Team operates freely throughout all areas of the incident site.

personnel, safety is a difficult task. This makes a Safety Officer essential on major incidents.

SAFETY OFFICER DUTIES

The Safety Officer's job is to monitor all phases of the operations and to advise the Incident Manager of procedures that reduce risk. This includes effective lighting, rest and relaxation schedules, vehicle traffic control, and utility shutdowns.

Safe operations complement scene control safety efforts. This includes proper lifting, patient securing techniques, and safe operations of tools and equipment. Use of protective equipment, such as breathing apparatus, headgear, and protective clothing, is an important factor. Personnel accountability is important in many mass casualty, fire, and law enforcement incidents. Infectious disease control is essential to ensure EMS personnel having direct patient contact are implementing proper precautions to protect themselves.

SAFETY OFFICER OPERATIONS

The Safety Officer should be an emergency services professional familiar with disaster operations. An individual with this background is well versed in Incident Management and communications procedures. The Safety Officer should also be familiar with nationally accepted safety standards. These standards include, but are not limited to:

1. OSHA Safety Standards—29 CFR, part 1910
2. National Fire Protection Association (NFPA) standard 1500—Fire Department Occupational Health & Safety Programs
3. NFPA 471, 472, 473—standards for Hazardous Materials Operations
4. NFPA 1521 Fire Department Safety
5. Infectious Disease Control Procedures (OSHA 29 CFR, part 1910.1030)

Safety Officers may be provided by non-medical agencies. Many urban fire departments have a full-time Safety Officer. Fire inspectors and/or training officers are qualified to serve in this capacity. Large EMS organizations may have a training officer with similar qualifications. Local and county governments have safety inspectors and risk management people who can provide safety expertise.

Specialized strike teams often have their own safety position. These safety specialists are not part of the Management Staff and do not have safety responsibility for the overall incident. Their duties are confined to the operations assigned to their team. This includes hazardous materials teams, high angle rescue teams, SWAT teams, confined space rescue teams, bomb disposal teams, heavy rescue teams, and underwater dive teams.

The Safety Officer should report to the Incident Manager upon arrival and receive an initial briefing. The Safety Officer is then responsible for monitoring safety procedures throughout the area and identifying any threats to personnel (scene threat assessment). In major disasters the Safety Officer may need support personnel to monitor several areas.

The Safety Officer should make corrections in procedures through the normal line of authority. Safety violations should be reported to the appropriate supervisors. There may be times when a serious safety violation warrants immediate action. THE SAFETY OFFICER SHOULD HAVE THE AUTHORITY TO STOP ANY OPERATION THAT IS LIFE-THREATENING TO PERSONNEL. Naturally, such action must have the moral support of the Incident Manager.

> **Critical Factor:**
>
> The Incident Manager is responsible for the safety of all personnel. In complex operations, a Safety Officer is needed to assist the Incident Manager.

LIAISON

One of the brutal lessons learned in the California wildfire experiences of the 1970s was that diverse agencies do not automatically cooperate. In day-to-day operations, each agency does its thing. Coordination is routine. In disasters, agencies that do not normally work together are thrown into a stressful and uncontrolled arena. Coordination is anything but routine. Operational goals differ, personnel do not know each other, terminology varies, and radio frequencies are incompatible. Under these conditions, coordination is a miracle.

These problems occur because many government public safety agencies operate as a closed system. In systems theory, a closed system is an organization that operates internally, with little input from, or exchange with, outside systems. An open system is the opposite. In an open system, the organization is structured to exchange information with other systems. Interaction between systems is sometimes referred to as "boundary spanning." This means that boundaries confining organizations are easily crossed.

It is vital that incident management systems operate as open systems. As an incident escalates, dozens of agencies may become involved. These agencies descend upon the command post with the greeting, "Hi, I'm here to help you" (pun intended).

The most effective means of coordinating with the outside world is through a Liaison Officer. The Liaison Officer serves as a link between the management system and outside systems or agencies. The Liaison Officer ensures "boundary spanning."

> **Critical Factor:**
>
> The Medical Incident Management System must coordinate with a myriad of outside agencies (open system). Liaison with outside agencies is a vital management function.

The Liaison Officer works with assisting agencies and cooperating agencies. An assisting agency is one that provides direct support and resources. This can include the EMS or medical agencies, law enforcement, fire departments, and public works. Cooperating agencies provide indirect support or service functions. Examples include utility companies, American Red Cross, advisory agencies (EPA, OSHA, etc.), and technical support agencies.

When an agency arrives at an incident, an agency representative is appointed. The representative must have authority to make decisions, represent the agency, and coordinate directly with the Liaison Officer. An agency representative provides a single point of contact for the Liaison Officer.

The primary function of the Liaison Officer is to funnel outside agency resources into the appropriate section of the EMS/IMS. Usually, assisting agencies function in the Operations Section. Cooperative agencies work in a support category under the Logistics Section or Planning Section. The Liaison Officer may receive requests from incident personnel for contacts with other organizations.

With multiple organizations, there is a potential for organizational conflict. We don't always get along. The Liaison Officer should try to identify possible conflicts between organizations. The Liaison Officer can serve as a mediator between conflicting agencies. Without liaison assistance, the Incident Manager often becomes involved in conflicts that misdirect his or her attention from more vital tasks.

WORKING WITH THE MEDIA

A mass casualty incident is a newsworthy event. But all too often the words "uh-oh, here comes the media," are uttered by members when operating at the scene. The arrival of media crews can be a major source of stress if you are not prepared to professionally and confidently address the issue.

Today's broadcast, print, or photo journalist is well-educated and informed regarding emergency incidents. Members of the media have to report back to an assignment editor with their story, and very often work under strict deadlines for presses rolling or live shots for the news. They need the story and/or their sound bite, and, if you don't give it to them, they'll get it from somewhere else.

We've all had the shock and dismay of reading the next day about an incident we worked and wondering if the reporter was at the same scene as we were. If a story is wrong, don't blame the reporter. Blame yourself. Ask the questions, "Did we cooperate with the media in every possible way? Did we give them the correct information?" If the answers are "no," an incorrect story is your fault or your organization's fault.

An Incident Manager needs a public information professional for media assistance. It's not possible to maintain the concentration and activity to manage an incident and conduct media briefings simultaneously. The media specialist designated in the Incident Management System is called the Public Information Officer (PIO) and is an integral member of the staff.

The topic of media relations could occupy one or more textbooks due to its specialization. In this text, the subject will be provided in the format of a brief overview.

> **Critical Factor:**
>
> Timely and accurate release of information in a professional manner is key to the positive reflection of your organization's action at the MCI. The command staff position of PIO is integral in EMS/IMS.

PUBLIC INFORMATION OFFICER DUTIES

In street language, the PIO's job description could read, "Keep the media off everybody's rear and make sure we look good." The PIO's job begins before the incident. A good PIO has already developed media contacts and a rapport with them that fosters trust, professional respect, and a willingness to attempt to work together. The media contacts get their story and the PIO makes the department look good. Not a bad trade off, eh? Most times in the local arena this goal is achievable. In many instances though, if your incident attracts national or international attention, the rapport with the local outlets may not be enough to get you through. On these occasions you might find yourself confronted with networks and reporters from around the world. In these cases the importance of a PIO on your command staff cannot be over emphasized. (See Figure 3-3.)

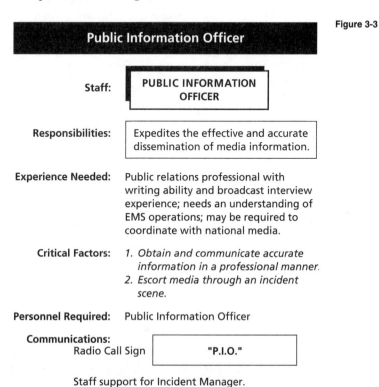

Figure 3-3

Public Information Officer

Staff:	PUBLIC INFORMATION OFFICER
Responsibilities:	Expedites the effective and accurate dissemination of media information.
Experience Needed:	Public relations professional with writing ability and broadcast interview experience; needs an understanding of EMS operations; may be required to coordinate with national media.
Critical Factors:	1. Obtain and communicate accurate information in a professional manner. 2. Escort media through an incident scene.
Personnel Required:	Public Information Officer
Communications: Radio Call Sign	"P.I.O."

Staff support for Incident Manager.

The PIO reports directly to the Incident Manager. The Incident Manager has the overall authority to authorize press briefings and the release of information. At large-scale or criminally related events, the release of information needs to be coordinated by all agencies involved in order to avoid compromise of patient confidential information or a criminal investigation. It is the obligation of the PIO to stay current with all pertinent data at the scene (units operating, present status of the incident, number of patients, types of injuries, hospitals that receive patients).

The PIO should establish a media briefing area separate from operational areas and the command post. Ideally, this area will provide the media with a good vantage point of the incident while ensuring their safety and crowd manageability. PIOs should also be prepared for requests for computer printouts, agency and incident fact sheets, incident maps and diagrams to assist the media. Release of this information is sometimes prohibited, so it is incumbent upon the PIO to be familiar with current departmental policy, governmental laws, and directives to ensure compliance.

The PIO should conduct scheduled incident briefings at predetermined and announced times. In many instances updates may be required between briefings due to major changes that might occur. Updates also facilitate the media contact with the Incident Manager and other staff members that operate at the scene. This control of access to the Incident Manager and responders allows the PIO to arrange interviews without compromising the incident operations.

News teams or reporters should not be permitted to roam freely throughout the operational area. This creates a safety hazard for them and an operational distraction to the working staff. All staff operating on the incident site should refer unescorted members of the media to the PIO and refrain from entertaining questions while they are engaged in patient care or rescue activities.

Broadcast crews go to great lengths to get close-up shots of scenes. As previously stated this can present great danger to them due to their lack of training and understanding of the dynamics of the particular scene. Some departments have embarked on a unique training program where members of the media are permitted to go through training programs that familiarize them with emergency operations, EMS patient care, firefighting, and rescue activities. This training program, permits the media participants to have controlled contact and experience with the tasks that we are exposed to everyday. Upon successful completion of this program, they are issued protective gear and a different colored press pass that allows closer access to the incident scene. This program has yielded a number of positive results for the department and the media.

1. The media now have hands-on experience with what they're covering and can report the actions of the scene more accurately, providing the sponsoring department with better coverage.
2. The media outlet obtains better positioning at the scene to get its story, while making the department look great.
3. An enhanced relationship between the department and the media is fostered, allowing the PIO and the department to hopefully obtain coverage when needed. The arrangement has been found to be a public administrative and media win-win.

4. Media tape footage can be accessed for operational critique and training purposes. In the event that your local laws do not permit this type of program and access, the PIO should arrange for the crews to be escorted through the safe and secure scene to assist them getting their shot.

Helping the media is helping your department. It gives you control, and helps to guarantee that the story is portrayed accurately. But most importantly, never lie or misrepresent the facts. Don't be afraid to say, "I don't know but I'll check that out and get back to you." Many years of work and rapport can be destroyed in a moment. The better coordination between public safety agencies and media, the better and more accurately informed the community will be during the emergency.

SUMMARY

The Management Staff consists of a Safety Officer, Public Information Officer, Liaison Officer, and Stress Management Team. As an incident escalates, the Incident Manager can appoint staff to assist command duties.

The Management Staff does not consist of medical professionals. Staff members are safety inspectors, public affairs professionals, liaison specialists, and stress management team members.

The job of the Management Staff is to assist the Incident Manager. The Liaison Officer interfaces with assisting agencies and cooperating agencies. Liaison keeps Incident Management an open system. The Safety Officer operates in all areas of the incident to ensure operations are conducted safely. The Trauma Intervention Team assists in maintaining the mental health and emotional well-being of incident workers. The Public Information Officer coordinates with the media and ensures the release of information.

CHAPTER QUESTIONS/EXERCISES

1. List several non-medical professionals in your area that could assist as members of a Management Staff.
2. Diagram the organizational structure of the Management Staff.
3. What are the functions of the Liaison Officer? What is a cooperating agency? Assisting Agency?
4. What are the duties of the Public Information Officer?
5. What is the Trauma Intervention Program concept? What type of individuals should participate on a Trauma Intervention Team?
6. What media relations programs are now in effect with public safety agencies in your area? How can these people be integrated into the IMS?

4

EMS OPERATIONS

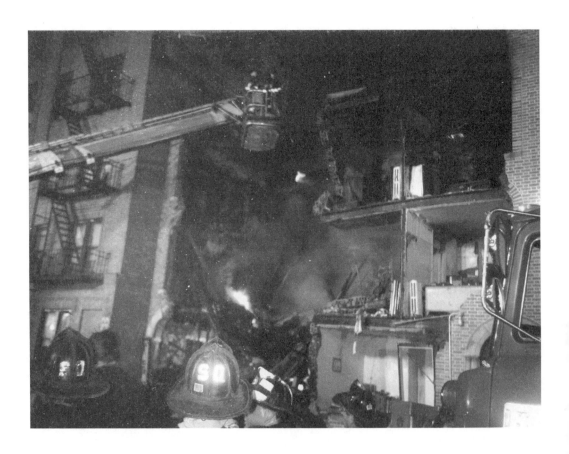

Chapter Objectives

After reading this chapter, you will be able to accomplish the following objectives:

1. Understand the concept of EMS operations.
2. Understand the relationship of operational functions to support functions.
3. Define the operations units in the EMS Incident Management System.
4. Define and discuss the effective use of medical strike teams and task forces.

WHAT ARE OPERATIONS?

Operations are direct, hands-on functions conducted by an organization to accomplish its mission. Most organizations are defined by their operational capabilities. For example, General Motors builds cars or Gateway makes computers. Both companies have extensive accounting systems and large research and development divisions. But you don't think of them in those terms. Their operations are the essence of the organization.

In the EMS Incident Management System, the treatment of patients is the mission. All the functions exist to support treatment operations. The Command Staff, the Logistics Section, and the Planning Section function to assist the Operations Section. (See Figure 4-1.)

Medical treatment operations involve triaging patients, treating them in logical order, and transporting them to a medical facility. To accomplish these treatment objectives, medical operations is divided into the following sectors:

1. Triage
2. Treatment (red, yellow, green)
3. Transport

EMS BRANCH DIRECTOR

The EMS Branch Director commands all operations units and serves directly under the Incident Manager. The EMS Director does not remain at a command post like the other section chiefs. The Branch Director is in the middle of the operational area. He/she has a moving position in the heat of the battle. (See Figure 4-2.)

The EMS Director has one of the busiest jobs on the incident scene. The Director is continually working with logistics and the staff to get scarce resources and support for EMS operations units.

It's extremely important to understand that the EMS Branch Director is a manager, and does not treat patients. It's hard for medical professionals to operate in treatment areas without "reaching out and touching someone." When a Director starts treating people, he/she is in big trouble, for no one is managing the bigger operational picture. In the operations area, good management ultimately leads to

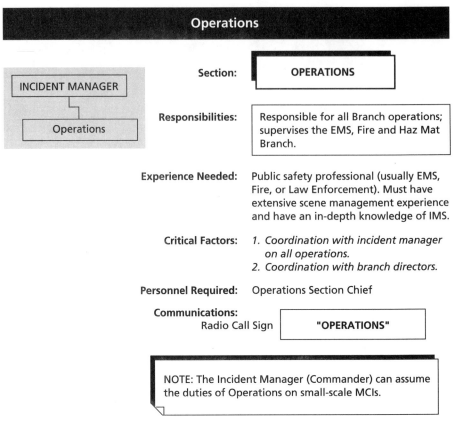

Figure 4-1

the saving of lives and limiting of suffering because it ensures that treatment personnel are adequately supported.

The EMS Branch usually has inadequate personnel and limited resources. A balancing act has to take place. Personnel must be rotated to where they are needed. If one treatment area gets real busy, people must be shifted.

The EMS Branch is also in close contact with the Logistics Section. Operations, at the early stages, will consume more supplies and equipment than Logistics can generate. Therefore, prioritizing supplies is as important as prioritizing personnel.

OPERATIONS/COMMAND RELATIONSHIPS

One of the most confusing aspects of any command system is the distinction between the Incident Manager and the Operational Branches. (See Figure 4-3.)

There is a tendency for Incident Managers to control operations and command responsibilities. This is especially true when the Incident Manager has an in-

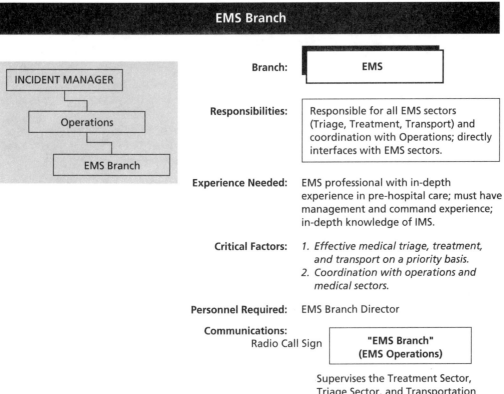

EMS Branch	
Branch:	EMS
Responsibilities:	Responsible for all EMS sectors (Triage, Treatment, Transport) and coordination with Operations; directly interfaces with EMS sectors.
Experience Needed:	EMS professional with in-depth experience in pre-hospital care; must have management and command experience; in-depth knowledge of IMS.
Critical Factors:	1. *Effective medical triage, treatment, and transport on a priority basis.* 2. *Coordination with operations and medical sectors.*
Personnel Required:	EMS Branch Director
Communications: Radio Call Sign	"EMS Branch" (EMS Operations)

INCIDENT MANAGER
Operations
EMS Branch

Supervises the Treatment Sector, Triage Sector, and Transportation Sector. Supervises Staging on major incidents.

Figure 4-2

depth background in operations. As an example, a medical professional, as Incident Manager, is tempted to command/control treatment operations. The same situation occurs in fire operations, when the fire commander attempts to control fire operations along with command responsibilities.

At routine incidents, command and operations are combined. Combining command and operations at major incidents is a mistake. As the incident escalates, operational demands begin to separate from management responsibilities. If the incident requires a command staff or other sections, such as Logistics or Planning, Management and Operations should be separated.

Critical Factor:

In an MCI, patient treatment operations should be separated from management responsibilities.

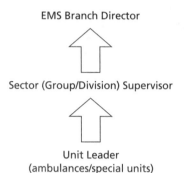

EMS Branch Director

Sector (Group/Division) Supervisor

Unit Leader
(ambulances/special units)

Figure 4-3 Operations Levels

THE SECTOR CONCEPT

Throughout this book there is emphasis on the flexibility of EMS/IMS. A Section can be separated into a Branch, such as the EMS Branch. The EMS Branch can be further divided into divisions or groups. (See Figure 4-4.)

A division is an element that operates in a specific geographical area. A group is a functional assignment that is not restricted to a specific area. Divisions relate to geography; groups relate to functions.

As an example, in a New York subway crash, New York EMS divided the Medical Branch into three divisions. There was a train division, which consisted of initial triage treatment, and extrication at the actual wreck. A platform division was established several hundred feet from the train. On the platform, patients were re-

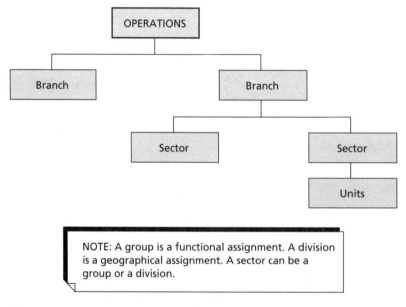

NOTE: A group is a functional assignment. A division is a geographical assignment. A sector can be a group or a division.

Figure 4-4 Branch Separation—National IMS Model

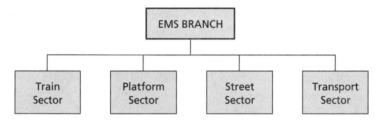

Figure 4-5 Dividing an Incident—Geographical Sectors

triaged, treated, and prepared for transport to the street level. A street division was formed at the station entrance (street level) for transport.

In many areas, groups/divisions are called sectors. The term "sector" began in urban fire ICS. Examples are a roof sector, an interior sector, or a basement sector. Many EMS systems also refer to sectors, such as treatment sector, triage sector, etc.

A disadvantage of sector terminology is that it does not distinguish between a geographical assignment and a functional assignment. The advantage of sector nomenclature is that it's simple; everything is a sector, instead of a group or division. In most cases, the term describing a sector is the important element. If you are assigned to a triage sector, you don't really care if it is a group or a division. (See Figure 4-5.)

For simplicity, the term "sector" will be used in this text. Where you see the words "group/division" in other literature, the term "sector" can be substituted.

Geographical sector assignments are usually made when the incident is separated into two or more areas. (Remember the example of the subway accident.) By assigning sectors, the EMS Branch Director effectively manages a complex incident. Let's consider more examples:

1. A bus accident with multiple injuries. Several casualties are in the bus, and several patients are outside the bus. Treatment operations may be divided into a bus sector and a street sector.
2. A high-rise fire (Floor 24). Casualties are on the 23rd floor. Treatment could be divided into sector 23 (to denote the floor), a lobby sector, and a street sector.
3. An airplane crash. The aircraft has broken into two sections, with patients on the runway. Treatment could be divided into a nose sector, a tail sector, and a runway sector.

Remember the toolbox analogy. Simple problems require few tools. When a problem becomes complex, the Incident Manager can dig into the toolbox and use whatever tools are necessary. Sectors are examples of these tools. Strike teams and task forces are also effective tools.

STRIKE TEAMS AND TASK FORCES

A strike team is a group of similar personnel or units under a single leader with common communications. Ambulances assembled for transport or five engine companies assembled for fire fighting are examples of strike teams. In each case, the units are assembled as a functional team. The team has communications, with the team leader reporting to the appropriate branch.

The task force is a group of dissimilar people or units temporarily assembled for a specific mission. A task force has a leader and common communications. Task force examples include an ambulance and two police units (medical/law enforcement), or a fire/rescue team working with an EMS Team.

Strike teams and task forces give the Operations Section Chief flexibility to accomplish any mission. It is impossible for planners to pre-determine every type of operational problem that may confront incident managers. By forming strike teams or task forces, problems can be solved according to needs.

Some task forces and strike teams are formed before an incident. This is common in the fire service with engine strike teams, or task forces consisting of two engines and a ladder company. Strike teams are not usually pre-established in EMS agencies. Most EMS teams remain as units and are assigned to sectors as appropriate.

Throughout an incident, strike teams and task forces can be formed and disbanded. Units and personnel can be assembled whenever they are needed. Their mission can last the duration of the incident or be completed in minutes. When a mission is finished, the strike team/task force personnel can be reassigned to their units to perform normal operations.

Actual examples demonstrate effective use of strike teams and task forces by operations commanders:

1. A military aircraft has crashed with munitions on board; there are numerous victims. An Explosive Ordinance Disposal (EOD) unit is combined with a medical unit to form a triage task force.
2. A mass shooting incident with numerous victims; the suspect's location is unknown. A SWAT unit is combined with a medical unit to form a treatment task force.
3. A tornado strike with major damage in three separate areas. EMS units are combined into strike teams and assigned to each area.
4. A building collapse with a critically injured trapped victim. A fire/rescue team is combined with an EMS team to form a rescue task force.

Critical Factor:

Personnel and equipment resources can be assembled into strike teams or task forces to accomplish specific missions. The task force/strike team concept gives managers flexibility to build operation teams as needs dictate.

SUMMARY

Operations are the identity of any organization. In a mass casualty incident, medical operations consist of triage, transport, and treatment.

Medical operations are under the command of the EMS Branch Director. This branch serves directly under the Operations Section Chief.

The EMS Branch Director is one of the busiest people at the incident. The EMS manager must move throughout patient treatment areas. His/her job is to ensure that adequate resources/supplies are available and that patients receive effective treatment. The Branch Director must coordinate resources needs with the Incident Manager.

A strike team is a group of similar units. A task force is a group of dissimilar units. Strike teams and task forces are operational groups that can be assembled to handle specific mission needs. This concept gives operational commanders flexibility. The most common element of EMS organization is the unit.

CHAPTER QUESTIONS/EXERCISES

1. Define the concept of operations in the EMS/IMS. What are the EMS operations units in the EMS Operations Branch?
2. What are the duties of the EMS Branch Director?
3. Briefly describe several cases where a medical professional should be the Operations Section Chief.
4. Define the terms "strike team" and "task forces."

5

EMS OPERATIONS FUNCTIONS

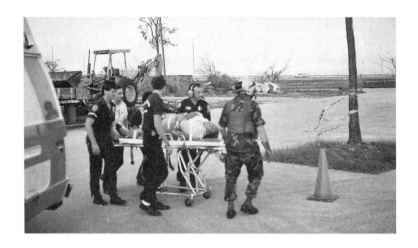

Chapter Objectives

After reading this chapter, you will be able to accomplish the following objectives:

1. Describe and diagram the units in the treatment sector.
2. Understand the relationship between treatment sectors and how this relationship affects patient flow.
3. Recognize triage as a management concept, and understand the importance of effective triage.
4. Understand the importance of transportation and the efficient use of scarce transportation resources.
5. Understand the importance of patient decontamination in today's chemical environment.
6. Define the duties of treatment sector supervisor and how they relate to the EMS Branch Director.

In Chapter 4, we discussed the Operation Section and its relationship to the Incident Manager and the Command Staff. In this chapter, we will break EMS operations into the sectors of treatment, triage, and transportation.

TRIAGE

Triage is a management issue. Specific triage techniques and protocols are discussed in Chapter 11.

A descriptive term for triage is "prioritizing." (Triage is a French word meaning "to sort.") When multiple patients are encountered, they must be prioritized. There are many analogies in other fields. In time management courses, students are encouraged to complete high priority projects first. (This is a method of time triage.) In business, given markets are prioritized, because all markets can't be reached. Target marketing is triaging the market. In medical triage, mass casualties are categorized, thus reducing large numbers of unmanageable patients into manageable groups. All patients can't be treated at once, so they are sorted, with the critical patients being treated first.

TRIAGE CATEGORIES

There are four patient categories. Each category is labeled by a descriptive term with an appropriate color.

RED—Immediate; immediate care is necessary or the patient will die. This category includes severe shock, airway problems, or depressed mental status.

YELLOW—Delayed; patient needs care, but is stable; patient could deteriorate to the immediate category. This category includes fractures, moderate bleeding, and minor shock.

GREEN—Minor; referred to as "walking wounded"; patients can treat their own injuries or wait many hours for treatment with no deterioration. This category includes minor fractures, minor lacerations or abrasions, and other minor injuries.

BLACK—Deceased. This category includes absence of vital signs, massive blood loss, very severe head injuries, and major chest trauma.

NOTE: The military and some civilian agencies use the term "expectant" to describe dead or dying patients. When we polled a group of medical professionals who were unfamiliar with the term, half of them thought it meant "expected to live." The term "expectant" is confusing and is not used in the IMS.

PATIENT ROUTING

Triage comes first in any incident without chemical contamination. In an MCI, triage is crucial. Upon arrival, first due units tend to start treatment. Finding the first critical patient and "working a code" is a serious mistake. It means other patients are not being sorted or triaged. More lives are saved by determining initial priorities, rather than treating the first patients encountered.

Picture the triage unit as a chute. Patients must flow through the chute before they enter a treatment area. When patients are scattered, triage teams must move quickly between patients. Patients are rapidly examined and marked by triage color. This is done with triage tags or colored vinyl tape. The color will determine what treatment area the patient is moved to or which patients are treated in place.

Patients who are brought to the medical team (casualty receiving area) physically pass through the triage "chute." This entrance area is marked by signs, scene tape, traffic cones, or all of the above. The triage unit serves as a traffic router that sets the treatment flow.

RE-TRIAGE

Triage is not a "done deal." A patient assigned a triage level is reassigned as conditions change. Treatment units should re-triage a patient while performing initial treatment. If the patient is re-triaged to a less severe level, treatment can be delayed. The team can move to a new patient. If a patient is deteriorating to critical, the proper treatment and transport protocols are administered. (NOTE: In some cases, re-triage may require a new triage tag.)

After treatment, a patient is re-triaged before transport to determine transport priority. Upon hospital arrival, the patient is triaged again. It is not unusual for a patient to be re-triaged four times from initial contact to hospital admission.

WHO DOES THE TRIAGE?

Does your highest-skilled or lowest-skilled treatment person perform triage? One school of thought says that triage is the most critical scene activity; therefore, the most skilled medical professional should do it. Another school believes that triage

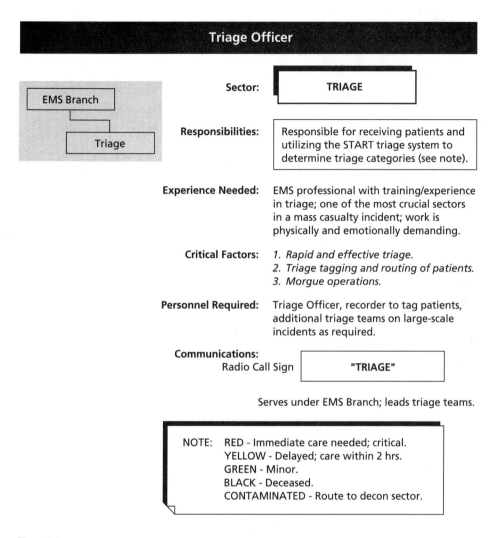

Triage Officer

EMS Branch

Triage

Sector: TRIAGE

Responsibilities: Responsible for receiving patients and utilizing the START triage system to determine triage categories (see note).

Experience Needed: EMS professional with training/experience in triage; one of the most crucial sectors in a mass casualty incident; work is physically and emotionally demanding.

Critical Factors: 1. Rapid and effective triage.
2. Triage tagging and routing of patients.
3. Morgue operations.

Personnel Required: Triage Officer, recorder to tag patients, additional triage teams on large-scale incidents as required.

Communications:
Radio Call Sign   "TRIAGE"

Serves under EMS Branch; leads triage teams.

NOTE: RED - Immediate care needed; critical.
YELLOW - Delayed; care within 2 hrs.
GREEN - Minor.
BLACK - Deceased.
CONTAMINATED - Route to decon sector.

Figure 5-1

should be simple, quick, and basic. Thus, an EMT or First Responder can triage, with trauma nurses, doctors, or paramedics treating critical patients.

Using BLS personnel with triage training is the most sensible approach. The purpose of triage is to get patients to critical care teams as needs dictate. Personnel with Advanced Life Support (ALS) skills need to be committed to patient stabilization, not to triage operations. (See Figure 5-1.)

BLS triage teams have less tendency to treat patients while performing triage. They tend to follow the basic steps of disaster triage, without complicating them. If they mis-triage a patient, the treatment team will find the mistake in its initial patient evaluation.

TRIAGE AT DISASTERS

As the number of patients increase, triage rules change. At routine incidents the best level of care is possible. There is a high ratio of EMS personnel per patient. If a patient has arrested, a long resuscitation effort is justified. Unless there are massive injuries, revival efforts are always attempted. There is rarely a black category of triage.

In an MCI or disaster, the situation changes. Resources are overwhelmed. There may be several patients per paramedic/EMT. A commitment of two or three medical professionals for a lengthy trauma code may result in several other critical patients dying. Therefore, the triage rules are different. If a patient has arrested due to trauma, he or she may be triaged as black. The crucial point is that triage rules change as incident levels change. In a routine medical incident, a high level of care is possible. In a medical disaster, austere care is the norm. Patients must be triaged accordingly.

KEY TRIAGE ISSUE

When conducting triage the EMS provider is confronted with a difficult task that is rarely subjected to frank discussion. Throughout our training we have been taught that the purpose of EMS is to save lives; but during the triage process, members may find themselves having to decide not to save a life because of massive injury and the number of other patients who require assistance. This decision results in "black tagging" a patient.

During the triage process a member must weigh a number of key factors (that are not fully defined or explained in most triage training programs) in order to execute a proper triage decision. A few key factors include total number of patients versus number of available resources (responders and ambulances), condition of patient being assessed, and local protocol mandates. Just because a patient may fit neatly into a "black tag" category should not automatically mean that he or she be written off as unsalvageable. Remember, triage protocols are guidelines established to assist the EMS provider in determining who gets treated first. If you have a patient who, under normal circumstances, you would attempt to resuscitate, and you have enough units operating on the scene to treat the total number of patients, then common sense should prevail and resuscitation should be commenced.

Local EMS providers are strongly encouraged to review this matter and to subject the topic to open and aggressive critique to determine what your agency policy should be.

TRIAGE STRESS

People who perform disaster triage for a lengthy period are often haunted by the experience. One EMT reported, "I triaged a 17-year-old girl as dead. I can still remember her wide open eyes."

Triage has sometimes been described as "playing God." Human beings have to make a determination of who is dead and who will be saved.

During a disaster, triage teams should be rotated with treatment teams. This limits an individual's exposure to the psychological/emotional trauma of triage. It also allows triage people to have the positive experience of patient treatment.

TIPS must be available to support triage personnel. A lengthy triage assignment should be followed by a TIPS defusing. Triage personnel should be further monitored after the incident by critical incident stress professionals. Incident Managers and EMS Branch Directors must consider the emotional toll of triage when making personnel assignments.

THE TREATMENT SECTOR

We're into Chapter 5 and finally down to the "nitty-gritty." Our system exists to effectively treat patients. The EMS Operations Section Chief or the EMS Branch Director (depending on the particular organizational structure) supervises the treatment sector. The treatment sector is divided into units based on triage categories. There are red, yellow, and green treatment teams.

In many instances the decision whether to treat in place or to establish a separate treatment area has spawned great discussions. As is the case with all other aspects of the Incident Management System, current conditions combined with common sense should be the prevailing factors when executing this decision. Just because we have many little boxes on the IMS chart is not a mandate to fill each one with a different person. For example, when we respond to a "garden variety" MCI, let's say a five-patient MVA, the person who is assigned the Triage Officer task will shift over to be the Treatment Officer once triage has been concluded. Another good example might be that once we have the finite number of units responding to the scene in our staging area, the Staging Officer can make a smooth transition to Transportation Officer. In most instances this transition occurs without problem. The goal of the IMS process is to maximize utilization of available resources to ensure effective and efficient operations, not to establish an unwieldy command structure.

In some cases the need to establish a separate treatment area becomes evident. Situations that present with numerous patients in a confined area most frequently require this decision. Other factors include, but are not limited to: presenting hazards to patient and rescuers, environmental issues such as inclement weather, and duration of operations and geographic obstacles that impact the ability of getting resources close to the incident. Once again, the emphasis on common sense and good incident assessment skills should be the overriding influences when making this determination.

The Treatment Officer answers directly to the EMS Branch Director and supervises all medical treatment units. (See Figure 5-2.) The treatment areas should be continuously evaluated for two important reasons:

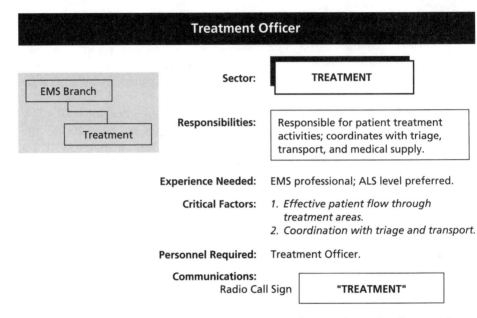

Figure 5-2

1. Treatment areas must be staffed to adequately handle patient flow.
2. Treatment areas must be properly supplied.

Ideally each treatment area should be staffed to handle the appropriate workload. In reality it's impossible to guess the staffing requirements. Therefore, treatment areas must be monitored. The yellow area may be overwhelmed, with the red area well staffed, or vice versa. Throughout the incident, needs in treatment areas may fluctuate. The Treatment Officer must shift personnel between treatment areas or contact the EMS Branch Director for more personnel.

The medical supply priority is the red treatment area. This unit will be consuming medications, I.V. fluids, oxygen, and trauma dressings at a high rate. The Treatment Sector Officer must ensure that medical supply demands are communicated to Operations so that Logistics can be contacted for supplies. It may be necessary to divert supplies from other areas to critical patients.

The Treatment Officer coordinates with Transportation. In a perfect script, patients should flow into a treatment area, be stabilized, and transported from the incident to a medical facility. In Murphy's world, patient backlogs develop in treatment areas. If patients are delivered to treatment areas faster than they are transported from the scene, a log jam develops. Treatment areas become "holding" areas.

In summary, the Treatment Officer is a person "in the middle." He/she must keep a balance of people in the treatment area and scream for more supplies and transportation.

RED TREATMENT UNIT

The red treatment unit performs emergency medical care for critical patients. (See Figure 5-3.) By definition, critical patients require immediate care and transport because of life-threatening trauma. Critical patients include general categories of shock, severe fluid loss, depressed mental status, and airway maintenance. (Specific treatment protocols and concepts will not be discussed.)

The key element in the EMS/IMS is an effective red treatment unit. Obviously proper triage and transport are needed to complement critical patient treatment.

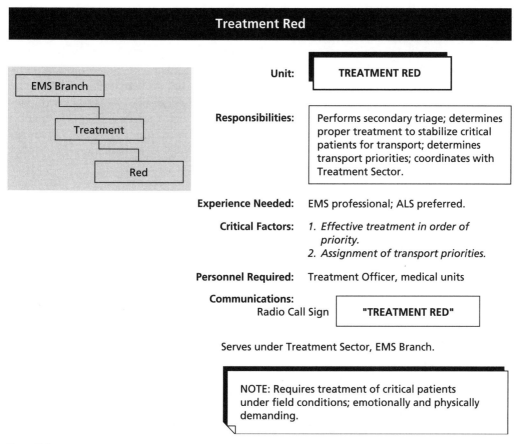

Treatment Red

EMS Branch
Treatment
Red

Unit: **TREATMENT RED**

Responsibilities: Performs secondary triage; determines proper treatment to stabilize critical patients for transport; determines transport priorities; coordinates with Treatment Sector.

Experience Needed: EMS professional; ALS preferred.

Critical Factors:
1. *Effective treatment in order of priority.*
2. *Assignment of transport priorities.*

Personnel Required: Treatment Officer, medical units

Communications:
Radio Call Sign   **"TREATMENT RED"**

Serves under Treatment Sector, EMS Branch.

NOTE: Requires treatment of critical patients under field conditions; emotionally and physically demanding.

Figure 5-3

> **Critical Factor:**
>
> All functions in the EMS Incident Management System exist to support the red treatment area. A breakdown in critical treatment and transport means that patients will die.

Medical professionals with the highest skill levels should be in the red treatment unit. This will include physicians, P.A.s, trauma nurses, and paramedics. It was mentioned that many of the IMS positions do not need medical staffing. Keep your best people out of staff positions; save them for critical treatment.

The equipment and supply requirements for the red treatment unit are demanding. This unit uses monitors, defibrillators, oxygen, suction, intubation equipment, and trauma dressings. The supply requirements include drugs, fluids, and infusion sets.

The red treatment unit is very stressful. There is usually a high patient flow, coupled with scarce supplies and equipment and a great deal of noise. In a disaster, multiple deaths can be anticipated in this treatment area. This area will contain biological hazards.

For these reasons, red treatment unit personnel need to be rotated and rehabilitated. This is not an area for a twelve-hour shift during an extended operation. The rehabilitation period requires rest, nourishment, and TIPS availability.

The red treatment unit leader is in command of the unit and coordinates with the EMS Branch Director or the Treatment Sector Officer. The information from the red treatment unit will usually involve supply/equipment needs, personnel requirements, and transportation needs. (This same type of information also applies to the yellow treatment unit.)

YELLOW TREATMENT UNIT

The yellow treatment unit treats patients classified as delayed. (See Figure 5-4.) These patients require treatment within hours to prevent deterioration to critical. The objective is to control the onset of shock, airway problems, and fracture stabilization. Patients in this category may have lacerations (without severe blood loss), fractures, blunt trauma, and moderate burns.

> **Critical Factor:**
>
> Patients in the yellow treatment area must be monitored to ensure they do not become critical.

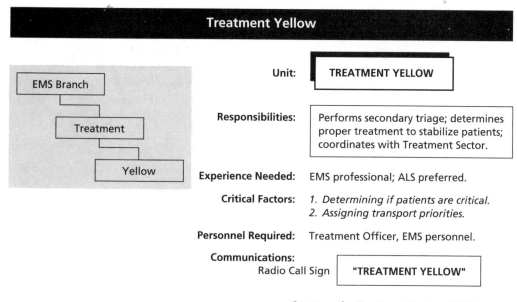

Treatment Yellow

| EMS Branch |
| Treatment |
| Yellow |

Unit: TREATMENT YELLOW

Responsibilities: Performs secondary triage; determines proper treatment to stabilize patients; coordinates with Treatment Sector.

Experience Needed: EMS professional; ALS preferred.

Critical Factors: *1. Determining if patients are critical.*
2. Assigning transport priorities.

Personnel Required: Treatment Officer, EMS personnel.

Communications:
Radio Call Sign | "TREATMENT YELLOW"

Serves under Treatment Sector, EMS Branch.

Figure 5-4

Patients enter the yellow treatment unit via triage. They can also flow from the red or green treatment units into the yellow area. Patients are transported from the yellow area to a medical facility. Although red patients have first priority in transport, yellow patients must also be considered. This is important if the patient's condition will become critical without intervention at a medical facility.

The yellow treatment unit is staffed by paramedics and trauma nurses, assisted by EMTs. In medical disasters, trauma physician support is helpful. (Remember that the red treatment unit gets physician priority.)

GREEN TREATMENT UNIT

The green treatment unit treats patients with minor injuries. (See Figure 5-5.) These patients almost triage themselves. They are walking, alert, and oriented. (Thus, the term "walking wounded.") These patients have minor lacerations, minor fractures, or blunt trauma. They have no airway or perfusion problems.

It is important in the green treatment protocol to immediately assess new patients, ensuring they are properly triaged. Patients who appear to have minor injuries may deteriorate into unconsciousness or a depressed mental state. Vitals may decline, forcing a triage re-classification. EMTs are suitable for green treatment operations.

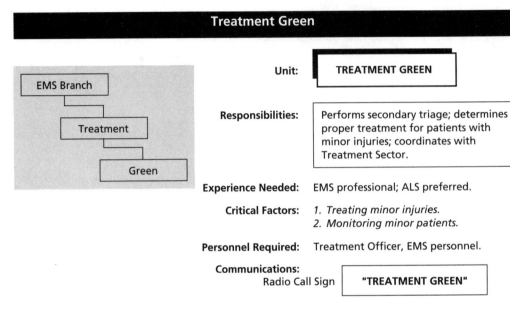

Figure 5-5

Supplies are not as critical in the green treatment area. Bandaging and minor splinting are commonly used supplies. There is no need for drugs, I.V. therapy, or oxygen. Patients in the green treatment category will eventually need medical care but are the lowest transport category.

MORGUE

The morgue area is for patients with no vital signs, and should be segregated from treatment areas and bystanders. If possible, a building, trailer, or truck should serve as the morgue. This area requires additional security to control entry. (See Figure 5-6.) Morgue activities must be coordinated with the law enforcement agency that has jurisdiction.

> **Critical Factor:**
>
> Patients in the morgue must be thoroughly examined and re-triaged.

Preservation of body parts, clothing, and valuables are necessary to assist in future identification. Naturally, personnel working in this unit will be severely

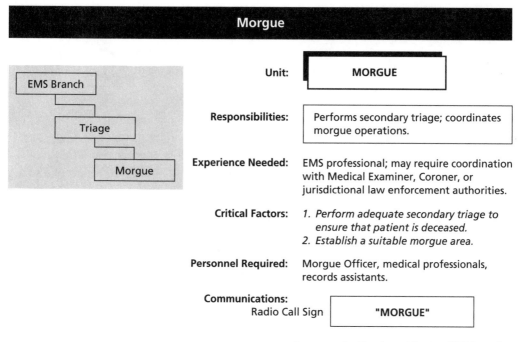

Morgue

Unit:	MORGUE
Responsibilities:	Performs secondary triage; coordinates morgue operations.
Experience Needed:	EMS professional; may require coordination with Medical Examiner, Coroner, or jurisdictional law enforcement authorities.
Critical Factors:	1. *Perform adequate secondary triage to ensure that patient is deceased.* 2. *Establish a suitable morgue area.*
Personnel Required:	Morgue Officer, medical professionals, records assistants.
Communications: Radio Call Sign	"MORGUE"

Serves under Treatment Sector, EMS Branch.

Figure 5-6

stressed. TIPs and clergy members should be assigned to assist. Personnel should be frequently rotated, with a tour of duty in this unit followed by a stress debriefing.

Funeral directors are helpful. Every disaster team should have a mortuary professional as a consultant. The National Association of Funeral Directors has a special unit called a D-Mort Team that is available to operate at major disaster sites. Unit members provide body preservation, identification, and assistance in handling grieving relatives.

TRANSPORTATION

In an MCI, transportation assets are overwhelmed in the early stages. The ultimate success depends on eventual treatment at a medical facility. This means that medical transportation, after initial treatment, is essential.

The transportation sector coordinates directly with the EMS Branch. (See Figure 5-7.) In an ideal situation (no MCI is ideal), patients flow from treatment areas to transportation vehicles and are immediately moved to a medical facility. In most MCIs, patients enter treatment areas faster than they are transported. There is a backlog of patients awaiting transport. As the patient bottleneck increases, transportation vehicles become a crucial element.

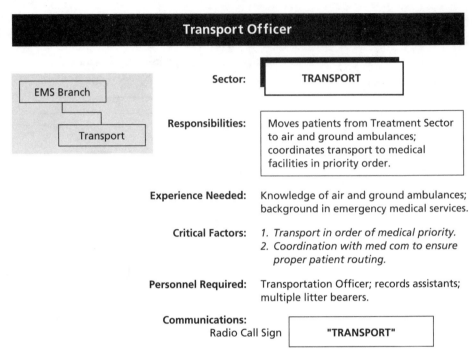

Figure 5-7

The transportation officer is responsible for securing transportation resources, maintaining transportation records, coordinating patient loading on a priority basis, and coordinating with Medical Control to determine receiving medical facilities.

TRANSPORTATION RESOURCES

In the IMS, transportation resources are categorized as air or ground assets. Ground transportation includes ambulances, buses, and private vehicles. Air units are helicopters or fixed-wing aircraft.

Ambulances are the most desired units. These vehicles have equipment and space for Advanced Life Support (ALS) treatment. A disadvantage is their inability to transport large numbers of patients. In an MCI, buses can be used to transport "walking wounded" patients. Whenever a bus is used, it should be followed by an ALS unit and have an ALS team on board. If any green patient "codes", or deteriorates, ALS is immediately available. Unfortunately, private vehicle transport is an uncontrollable factor in many MCIs. Well-meaning citizens and law enforcement officers transport victims in their cars to the nearest medical facility. This usually happens before medically trained personnel establish the IMS.

Patients transported by private vehicle are frequently "horror stories." Patient records are non-existent. They are not triaged or properly treated. Patients become lost because of removal without the knowledge of on-scene professionals. They are often taken to the wrong facility. Transport by personal vehicles should cease as soon as the IMS is established. Law enforcement officers should be trained to refrain from transporting patients.

Case histories show that in many MCIs, medical centers near the incident have been filled with privately transported patients. Medical facilities must notify Medical Control when such patients arrive. Transport Officers may be unpleasantly surprised to find a critical trauma center is full before the first "official" patient is transported.

Air transport is usually restricted to helicopter operations. Helicopters can transport over long distances without traffic or terrain restrictions. Establishing a safe and effective landing zone (LZ), also called a helspot, is the responsibility of the transportation sector. Helicopters require an approach free of obstructions, a safe landing area, proper signals, lighting, and fire units at the LZ.

Establishing a helspot at the immediate incident site may not be possible. This means patients must be transported by ground vehicle to the LZ, with coordination between the transportation officer and the LZ. To establish such coordination, the officer can reach into the IMS toolbox and establish a helicopter strike team.

Because of the need for runways, fixed-wing aircraft transportation is seldom a factor in an MCI. In a medical disaster, the National Disaster Medical System (NDMS) plan calls for the establishment of regional evacuation points near major airport runways. This is limited to full-scale catastrophic events; MCIs do not generate a patient load that justifies mass transport via fixed-wing aircraft.

TRANSPORTATION COORDINATION WITH IMS ELEMENTS

The Transportation Officer cannot realistically perform all the duties discussed. He/she must use incident management tools for help. Two areas that require coordination are obtaining transport units and coordinating transportation with medical facilities.

In an MCI, Transportation can directly obtain transport vehicles. In a disaster, this responsibility must be delegated. Large numbers of units are needed. These units will be called in "waves." Coordinating these resources will overwhelm the transportation officer.

Another critical transportation issue is determining which medical facilities are to receive which patients. In an MCI, the nearest medical facilities may be overwhelmed, and other facilities may be underutilized. Key issues are the location of local/regional hospitals, available bed space, ICU capabilities, ER size, physician availability, and specialties such as surgical units, burn units, or pediatrics.

The Transportation Officer operating in the hysteria of the field cannot personally process or keep track of the issues just discussed. In the IMS, this information is maintained by Medical Control. (Medical Control will be covered in Chapter 7.)

Many disaster plans call for hospital status to be maintained by a communications center or a medical control center (usually a hospital). The important point is that medical facility status and availability are not coordinated by a harassed on-scene manager. Instead, hospital status is delegated to a communications center or a medical control center.

Without delegation, a Transportation Officer must call for transportation vehicles, stage the vehicles, and decide which patients will go to which medical center. (See Figure 5-8.) This is in addition to coordinating with triage to keep patients flowing into the treatment areas, and transporting patients to ambulances after initial treatment. This is all done on the run, with a clipboard in one hand and a portable radio in the other.

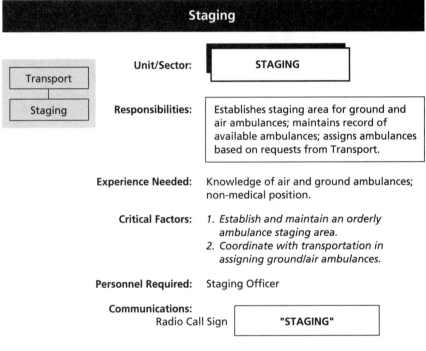

Figure 5-8

By delegating functions to Medical Control, the picture is different. A quick radio call from the Transportation Officer to Medical Control gets an update on bed availability and facility status. When ready to transport, the Transportation Officer learns from Medical Control where to send the patients.

MULTIPLE CASUALTY INCIDENT (MCI) GUIDE

First Arriving Unit
- Conduct initial assessment of incident, size, site, and hazards
- Establish command post
- Request additional units if needed
- Initiate primary triage
- Direct arriving EMS personnel to appropriate areas

Triage Sector
- Implement triage system S.T.A.R.T. and affix triage tags to patients
- Report progress and needs to EMS Command Officer
- Limit treatment to:
    positional airway management
    severe hemorrhage control
    shock by position
- Move patients by priority to Treatment Sector

Treatment Sector
- Limit access of non-essential personnel
- Obtain police assistance in securing perimeter
- Establish sector close to incident and accessible to vehicles
- Re-triage patients on arrival
- Group patients by priority
- Limit medical care to urgent needs

Transport Sector
- Transport by medical priority
- Track patients and hospital destination information
- Request availability status:
    Area hospitals
    Specialty referral centers
- Distribute patients evenly to avoid hospital overloading
- Don't overload a facility—this impacts on 9-1-1

Staging Sector

- Establish sufficient distance from incident
- Don't gridlock units
  - Have Staging Sector Officer retain keys to vehicles
  - Provide best access and egress routes to dispatcher
  - Request police department assistance, if necessary, to secure area
  - Track inventory of units arriving at site and relay to EMS Branch Director

The importance of proper action by the first due unit cannot be overstressed. In a major MCI, the ratio of patients to first due providers could be ten to one, twenty to one, or more. Attempting to immediately treat patients is not a prudent course of action. Two functions must take precedence: management and triage.

The officer or senior member is the Incident Manager. He or she is responsible for all IMS functions, and only has one or two other members to be assigned. The other member(s) must be immediately assigned to triage. (The unit should have a triage kit that includes triage tags/ribbons, a checklist, and triage vests.) The triage assignment should be made as soon as it is discovered that there are mass casualties.

The first due Incident Manager must communicate patient estimates and ask for help. The estimate will rarely be accurate, but the objective is to let the "world" know the gravity of the situation. The Incident Manager must also communicate the command post location (he/she *is* the command post) to the communications center, and remain at the command post until relieved.

These steps are logical but can be emotionally difficult. They require a medical responder to temporarily forgo a treatment role and, instead, assume a management role. If you find yourself treating a patient, you and the remaining patients are in real trouble because there is no Incident Manager "minding the store." Remember: Grab your radio (not your trauma box), make an educated guess about the patient numbers, and call for help. Lastly, make sure you get feedback. On a high-radio traffic day, the communications center could miss your radio call.

Consider an example. You respond to a construction accident. The caller says, "Someone is hurt." On arrival, you see a large section of the building collapsed, with people running all over the place. At least three victims can be seen. You yell, "Triage!" to your partner. The foreman is visibly shaken and tells you there are ten workers in the collapse zone. You key your mike and state calmly, "Rescue ten to EMS, emergency traffic; we have an MCI building collapse; estimate fifteen patients; that is one-five patients. Request three additional ambulances and heavy rescue. The command post will be at Bader Avenue and Woodham Street." You then remain at the command post waiting for other units, and assign them to triage and treatment functions as needs dictate. You remain the Incident Manager until a senior officer/manager arrives.

SUMMARY

Key elements in the Operations Section are triage, treatment, and transportation.

Triage is a major patient management concept. It involves a preliminary examination to determine which, if any, patients require immediate treatment. These are immediate (RED) patients. Delayed (YELLOW) patients need care within two hours to prevent deterioration into the critical category. Minor (GREEN) patients do not require high levels of medical treatment. Patients who are dead, or near death and untreatable, are classified as BLACK and sent to a separate area.

As patients are moved from triage, to treatment, to transport, they are continually re-triaged. This ensures that the patient has not moved into another treatment category.

The essence of IMS is the effective treatment and stabilization of our patients. The treatment sector is the element that treats disaster victims. Treatment areas are divided and color coded according to the triage categories. Immediate (RED) patients are the highest treatment priority. Delayed (YELLOW) patients require stabilization to prevent them from becoming critical. Minor (GREEN) patients require the lowest level of treatment. These patients are often called "walking wounded."

The treatment units, especially RED, consume large amounts of medical supplies. In most disasters, supply depletion is a grim reality. The treatment units must closely coordinate with the supply unit in the Logistics Section.

The transportation unit is responsible for on-scene patient flow from triage to treatment, and from treatment to transport vehicles. The transportation unit must also coordinate patient transport with the appropriate medical facilities and maintain records of where patients were transported.

The Transportation Officer may have to delegate responsibilities on large incidents and upgrade from a unit to a sector. Vehicle appropriation and vehicle status can be accomplished via Medical Control. Medical Control can be a communications center or medical facility. A staging unit, ground units, and air units are elements of a Transportation Sector.

CHAPTER QUESTIONS/EXERCISES

1. Diagram the units in the treatment sector. Define each unit function.
2. Define triage. Discuss the management aspects of triage.
3. List and define the four major triage categories.
4. What are the duties of the Transportation Officer?
5. List the immediate transportation assets in your community (air and ground). What regional transportation vehicles are available?
6. Define staging. What is the role of the staging concept in MCI operations?
7. You are in charge of the first arriving unit in a twenty-casualty MCI. What are your immediate duties? What responsibilities should be delegated to your partner?

6

EMS LOGISTICS

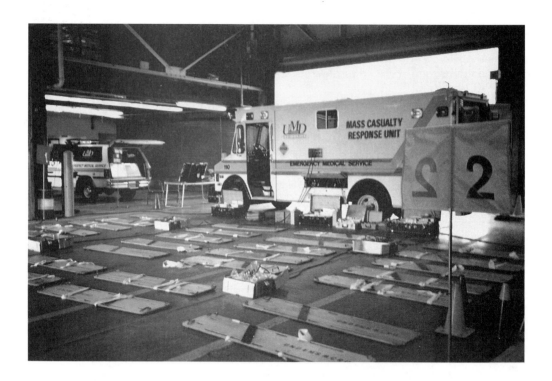

Chapter Objectives

After reading this chapter, you will be able to accomplish the following objectives:

1. Define the critical functions of logistics in relation to operations support.
2. List the duties of the Logistics Section Chief, and how he/she relates to the Incident Manager.
3. Discuss medical supply concepts including the "push versus pull" theory and the "cache concept."
4. Describe the functions of the facilities unit.
5. Describe the functions of the security unit.
6. Identify critical points in a logistics plan.

In Chapter 4, Operations was defined as the essence of an EMS organization, the medical treatment of patients. Operations needs support. Without supplies and communications, Operations is ineffective. This essential support function is provided by Logistics, or the Logistics Section in the IMS. The Logistics Section consists of the Logistics Section Chief, the medical supply unit, the communications unit, the facilities unit, and the security unit. (Communications will be discussed as a complete chapter.)

LOGISTICS SECTION

"Operations to Logistics; we need more supplies" is a familiar radio transmission in any MCI. In a regional disaster (a big earthquake or hurricane), supplies may arrive by the truckload or planeload. Consumption will still exceed distribution. Personnel support is closely related to supply support. Disaster team members will need food, water, shelter, rehabilitation, and security.

In small incidents, the Incident Manager can directly handle the logistical needs. As the incident escalates, supplies rapidly diminish. The early establishment of a medical supply unit is second only to establishing operations personnel.

> **Critical Factor:**
>
> A mass casualty incident will consume supplies on responding units; a medical disaster will deplete regional supplies.

In major incidents, a Logistics Sections Chief must be appointed. The Logistics Section Chief must coordinate with the EMS Branch Director and the Management Staff. Because of high clerical and communications demands, Logistics must work in a quiet and controlled area. Incident operations areas are too noisy and chaotic. In Logistics, clipboards, laptop computers, hand-held radios, and telephones are the tools. (See Figures 6-1 and 6-2.)

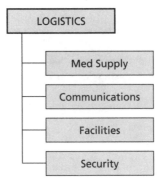

Figure 6-1 The Logistics Section

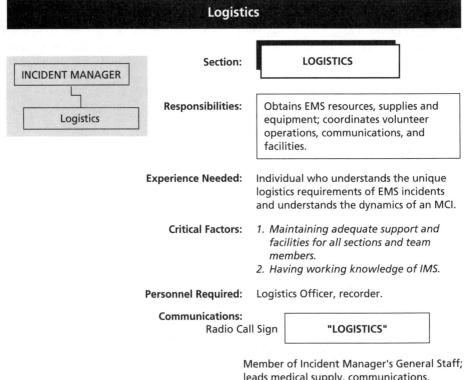

Figure 6-2

EMS SUPPLY UNIT

Diminishing supplies is a concept synonymous with disaster operations. Supplies are materials and medications that are consumed and cannot be reused. Equipment, in some cases, can be moved from one patient to another; supplies cannot.

Supplies are listed in several categories. (Detailed supply lists are in medical texts.) Drug supplies are the medications, including oxygen, carried by ALS Units. I.V. supplies include fluids and infusion sets. Personal Protection Equipment (PPE) includes gloves, masks, goggles, gowns, and disposal bags. Bandaging materials are classified as supplies. Equipment that cannot be transferred between patients should be considered as supplies. This includes cervical collars, backboards, and splints.

Initially, supplies come from responding units. A call for additional supplies is made by the Incident Manager. If supply levels are taxed, a Medical Supply Officer should be appointed to appropriate more supplies. (See Figure 6-3.) In an MCI, a

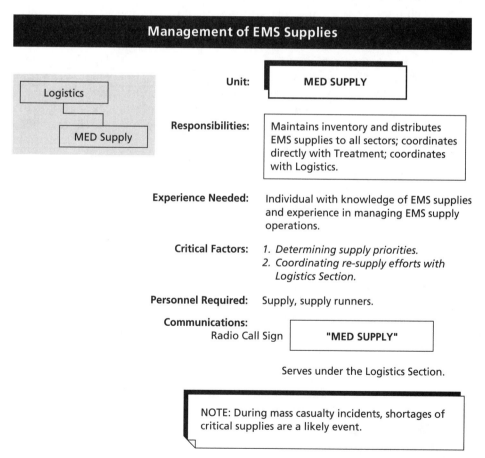

Management of EMS Supplies

Logistics
MED Supply

Unit: **MED SUPPLY**

Responsibilities: Maintains inventory and distributes EMS supplies to all sectors; coordinates directly with Treatment; coordinates with Logistics.

Experience Needed: Individual with knowledge of EMS supplies and experience in managing EMS supply operations.

Critical Factors:
1. *Determining supply priorities.*
2. *Coordinating re-supply efforts with Logistics Section.*

Personnel Required: Supply, supply runners.

Communications:
Radio Call Sign | **"MED SUPPLY"**

Serves under the Logistics Section.

NOTE: During mass casualty incidents, shortages of critical supplies are a likely event.

Figure 6-3

medical supply unit (probably one person) will be adequate. A full Logistics Section is rarely needed.

In large operations, the Medical Supply Officer may need help. This could include a recorder to maintain records and runners to unload and transport supplies to the treatment areas. If supply problems escalate, a Logistics Section Chief is needed. Supply appropriations may become statewide or national.

People with a medical supply or medical purchasing background are excellent sources for the medical supply unit. Medical treatment professionals should not serve in this unit. They shouldn't "wear themselves out" in the non-treatment areas.

THE "PUSH-PULL" CONCEPT

A disaster area is supplied using the push or pull method. In a pull supply system, field units order supplies as needed. This system has disadvantages. First, effective communications are essential for the system to function. If you can't talk to someone, you can't go supply shopping. Second, the pull system is slow to react. There is a lag time from order to arrival. When you get supplies, you need more. The advantage is a "tailor made" order (time permitting). If you need unusual supplies in type or quantity, they can be specified.

In a push supply system, pre-determined supplies are forwarded to the disaster scene. (They are pushed.) The supply needs of many disasters are predictable. For example, in an airplane crash, a large percentage of burns, lacerations, and fractures can be expected. Based on the number of survivors, I.V. fluids, backboards, splints, and trauma dressings are automatically pushed to the scene in the appropriate quantities.

The push system is a military logistics concept. The success of Operation Desert Storm was attributed to effective logistics. Supply needs were anticipated and stored in forward areas. When the ground offensive began, fast moving units found fuel, water, and ammunition waiting at critical locations. It was an ingenious push operation.

EMS and fire department operations are based on a push system. Vehicles are equipped and supplied for a predictable day. This works about 360 days per year. Some days are bad, and on-board supplies are not enough. An outside push to resupply the unusual incident is needed. Since a push is based on a prediction, the pushed supplies are not exact. If there are shortages, on-scene units can pull the extra supplies via radio. In summary, the system is lots of push, with a little pull. Make an educated guess, overestimate for a safety factor, and go for it.

Critical Factor:

Develop a "push" supply system by storing medical supply caches at key locations.

DISASTER CACHES

A cache is a store of equipment or provisions. A disaster cache is a store of predetermined supplies and equipment that can be immediately "pushed" to a disaster scene.

An ideal cache configuration is two large cases, sandwiched between several backboards. Typical cache supply lists are included in Figure 6-4. A cache is sealed and contains non-perishable supplies. Disaster caches can be kept at key locations throughout a city, county, or region. In an MCI or disaster, a cache can be loaded into a vehicle and "pushed" to the scene.

Fluid caches preferably should be kept in hospitals and rotated into the normal supply system. "Fresh" fluids are always available, and shelf life dates are not exceeded. This is fiscally responsible and medically sound. Several cases of fluids can be "pushed" to satisfy I.V. needs.

The following example demonstrates a "push-pull" supply system and disaster caches:

> An airplane crashes on landing. There are 90 passengers; 50 are alive. First arriving units describe the scene and give a rough patient estimate. Two disaster caches and two fluid caches are transported. This is based on logistical standing orders (Logistics protocol). During treatment operations, burn cases are not as high as anticipated. Only one fluid cache is used. However, the Treatment Officer discovers that a large number of children are involved. Pediatric cache supplies are not adequate. The Logistics Officer orders additional pediatric splints.

NOTE: Airports are required to maintain a large supply of mass casualty equipment such as backboards, BLS supplies, etc. These supplies can be integrated into an MCI protocol.

In this incident, the pushed supplies account for 95% of the logistics needs. The additional supplies are pulled. Most importantly, patient needs are met with adequate supplies. The system works based on planning.

Basic life support (BLS) public disaster kits should be placed in communities vulnerable to large-scale natural disasters. This especially applies to hurricane, tornado, or earthquake regions.

Immediately after Hurricane Andrew, fire stations were inundated with patients. (The phones were out, so people drove to the nearest firehouse.) One fire station reported 400 people seeking medical help. BLS supplies were consumed immediately.

Placing community disaster kits in fire stations, schools, and shelters ensures a dispersal of basic supplies. These kits can also be transported to smaller disasters, like an airplane crash or tornado. Disaster kits allow public assembly locations to be self-sufficient for BLS treatment.

The basic supplies needed in a disaster kit are listed in Figure 6-5. Plastic storage boxes, available at discount stores, make excellent containers. The containers can be shrink wrapped to seal and waterproof the container. A source of body bags and refrigerated storage should be identified in an MCI Logistic Plan.

Figure 6-4 Okaloosa County EMS—MCI Supply Cache

	BOX 1
2 Bag (12) ct	Bandage—Elastic flexicon 4″
12 Bag (12) ct	Bandage—Kerlix 4″
2 Box (25) ct	Bandaid
24	Bandage, triangular
24	Dressing, Vaseline 3 × 9
6 box (25) ct	Gauze sponge—sterile 4 × 4
12	Ice pack—instant
1 box (20) ct	Bulk dressing
6	Eye pads
20	Burn sheets
12	Tape, adhesive 1″
12	Tape, adhesive 2″
1 box (100) ct	Alchohol wipes
6	Stethoscope
6	Adult bp cuff
1	Large adult bp cuff
1	Child bp cuff
4	Saline, 1000cc irrigation
6	Rescue shears
4	Flashlights
4 sets	Batteries
5	Multi-trauma pak
5 (100) ct	Gloves, disposable, large
5 (100) ct	Gloves, disposable, medium
12	Emergency thermal blanket

	BOX 2
12	Ice pack, instant
2	Airway, size 0
4	Airway, size 3
4	Airway, size 5
17	Cervical cardboard headbed
11	Cervical collars—size no neck
6	Cervical collars—regular
6	Cardboard splints—18″
6	Cardboard splints—24″
2	V-vac suction
2	V-vac replacement cartridge
2	Oxy nasal cannula
12	Adult oxy mask, non-rebreather
5 (100) ct	Gloves, disposable, large
5 (100) ct	Gloves, disposable, medium
2	Oxy manifold sys 6 outlets
1	Oxy K cyl adapter for E type
1	Oxy regulator, D cyl
1	Oxy hose, 10 feet
1 set	Treatment area flags
1 set	IMS vests
2 set (125) ct	Triage ribbons

Figure 6-5 Okaloosa County Emergency Management

PUBLIC DISASTER KIT	
5	4 × 4 PACKS
20	Multi-trauma dressings
24	Ace bandages
24	Triangular bandages
4	Kling packs
1	Tape, 1″ box of 12
1	Tape, 2″ box of 12
1	Bandaids, box of 200
1	OB kit
2	Abdominal pads, box of 20
1	Gloves, large (box)
1	Gloves, medium (box)

Critical Factor:

Distribute public disaster kits in regions vulnerable to mass disaster.

Larger disaster caches are used by regional or national disaster teams. They are usually stored in disaster trailers or trucks. The caches can be quickly palletized for shipment on helicopters or fixed wing military aircraft. These caches can treat a hundred patients or more.

The treatment supplies in large caches should be kept in storage boxes capable of being carried by one person. The supplies and equipment are categorized as red, yellow, or green. Red supplies are for critical care treatment and include ALS medical and trauma equipment. Yellow supplies include materials for intermediate care patients. Green boxes include BLS supplies for the walking wounded patients.

The boxes are color coded to indicate treatment areas. By this method, treatment areas are quickly established. With three or four red boxes in the red area, you're ready to go. Anyone who isn't color blind can be the supply runner.

Figure 6-4 provides examples of supplies carried in treatment caches by disaster medical assistance teams (DMAT). These supplies are not all-encompassing and exclude medications. Other supplies and equipment that complement a large disaster cache are backboards, folding stretchers (military type), oxygen cylinders, and blankets.

The large disaster cache system was effective during Hurricane Andrew and Hurricane Iniki. In Chapter 12, Hurricane Andrew supply operations are discussed in detail.

COMMAND CACHES

Management operations have logistical needs like medical operations. During routine incidents, command does not use significant material. In an MCI, administration materials and supplies are needed to operate the command system.

A command cache has the following materials:

1. Reflective command vests with bold lettering to identify command positions.
2. Patient treatment forms.
3. A manual of standard operating procedures, medical protocols, resources, and support agencies.
4. A Plexiglas or plastic laminated checklist for each position.
5. Grease pencils or Sharpe weatherproof markers.
6. Treatment flags (red, yellow, green) to mark treatment areas.
7. GPS receiver (for helicopter landing zones).
8. Flashlights/strobe lights.
9. Vinyl tape (red, yellow, green).
10. Cyalume chemical light sticks (red, yellow, green).

A large plastic container labeled "command cache" should be kept in a command or supervisor's vehicle. In a regional or national disaster, command caches are transported with the disaster caches. The command cache is used first. Vests and checklists are distributed, and treatment areas are marked as a first step.

The command cache is an inexpensive and effective method of establishing scene management early. Management tools are deployed as fast as the medical tools.

FACILITIES

The facilities unit provides living facilities, food, and water for on-scene personnel. (See Figure 6-6.) Normal short-term incidents do not require a facilities unit. In a long-term incident, such as an MCI or disaster, facilities for personnel are required. Facilities are similar to supplies and equipment; they are taken for granted until needed.

Facility support in many incidents is provided by volunteer organizations like the American Red Cross and the Salvation Army. This support consists of portable canteens that provide food and beverages. Local fast-food franchises in the pizza and hamburger industry provide mass feeding as a donation.

Support organizations are a key element in disaster plans. Local emergency management agencies are the usual source for such plans. Your local emergency manager can implement support agreements with non-profit and business organizations for on-scene facilities and food. (See Chapter 9.)

Facility functions can be delegated to the emergency management agency. Medical personnel should not be used for facility operations.

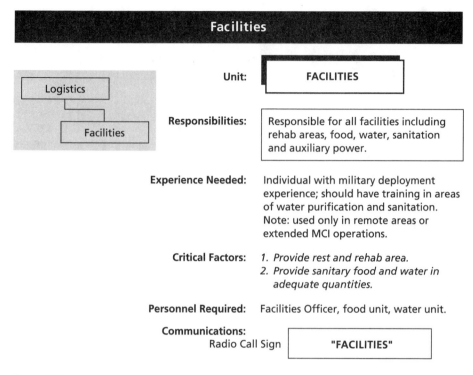

Figure 6-6

Adequate site facilities also function as a rest and rehabilitation area for working personnel on long-term incidents. This area is called REHAB in many fire incident management systems. Rest and relaxation, even for a few minutes, can reduce stress and crew fatigue. A granola bar and a glass of Gatorade, in a quiet area, is worth its weight in gold.

SECURITY

In the national IMS model, the security unit operates in the Logistics Section. In the EMS Incident Management System, the Incident Manager should make an early scene threat assessment and assign security functions to the appropriate law enforcement agency.

A law enforcement official may be the Incident Manager or share a unified command position with a fire commander. This structure applies to incidents like a barricaded suspect with hostages, a mass shooting, civil disturbance, or terrorism. In these instances, the EMS Operations Branch is structured as in any other MCI or disaster. The concern is protection of medical personnel from gunfire.

Security issues pertinent to IMS are:

1. Traffic control—major concern on most incidents; need to coordinate with the Incident Manager to ensure that streets are blocked or traffic diverted to provide a safe rescue and treatment area.
2. Treatment area security—treatment areas should have controlled entry; in incidents where large numbers of children are involved, especially schools, it may not be possible to keep distraught parents from treatment areas.
3. Morgue area—security is essential; keeping friends or relatives out of this area is difficult; emotional care is a major concern.
4. Medical disaster—major regional incidents may require U.S. Marshall, National Guard or military security; for example, in Hurricane Andrew, Army and National Guard security were assigned to all disaster teams.
5. Terrorism—there may be a secondary explosive device (binary weapon) designed to kill or injure emergency personnel.

In summary, security is a concern at all EMS incidents. It is coordinated with the command post and assigned to law enforcement or military professionals.

KEY LOGISTICAL POINTS

1. Develop a logistics plan—write supply estimates for an MCI and medical disaster; establish sources of medications and fluids; draft written communications procedures for pulling extra supplies; consider supply needs in budgets.
2. Coordinate with emergency management in identifying support agencies—develop a facilities support plan with support agencies and businesses; identify mutual aid agencies that can provide logistics; implement mutual aid agreements or memorandums of understanding (MOU) with support agencies.
3. Identify and train medical supply personnel—issue checklists and vests to supply/logistics personnel; include logistics personnel on emergency call rosters.
4. Set up disaster caches—store supplies in portable cases at key locations; have a protocol to automatically push caches to a major incident; store public disaster caches at fire stations, shelters, and public buildings; implement a disaster trailer for regional medical disasters.
5. Establish caches for mass decontamination from a chemical-biological terrorist incident. (See Chapter 8.)
6. Test logistics—conduct supply drills by calling for supplies at hypothetical locations; realistically simulate supply capabilities during mass disaster exercises.

Critical Factor:

Simulate logistics problems and test logistics operations during disaster exercises.

SUMMARY

EMS operations require intense logistics support. The Logistics Section includes the medical supply unit, the communications unit, the facilities unit, and the security unit.

Medical disasters can quickly deplete supplies. On routine incidents, the Incident Manager can handle the logistical needs. In an MCI, a medical supply unit must be established if supply demands overwhelm the system. In a disaster, a full Logistics Section will be needed.

Supply requirements in an MCI are based on experience. These pre-determined supplies are transported to an incident scene. This is a push supply system. If additional supplies are required, they can be ordered (pulled). An effective logistics procedure is to have pre-stocked supplies available for immediate transport to ensure a workable "push" system.

Pre-arranged supplies are called disaster caches. Caches are stored at key locations for a rapid and efficient supply push to a disaster scene. Large plastic storage boxes or cases are used. Disaster caches may be stored in response trailers or disaster vans for regional or national disasters. BLS supplies should be stored in fire stations and public shelters in earthquake and hurricane regions. These caches are public disaster kits.

Command and administration supplies are needed to operate the IMS. These materials are stored in a command cache for effective deployment. Command supplies include identification vests, reference materials, checklists, and supplies for working in treatment areas and helicopter landing zones.

Long-term incidents require a facilities unit. This unit provides food, shelter, and rehabilitation. The local emergency management agency, with public support agencies such as the Salvation Army or American Red Cross, is the best means of establishing a facilities unit.

Terrorist incidents also place high demands on security. Security is a logistics function in the national IMS model. In most disaster incidents, security is provided by local and regional law enforcement agencies. Security functions are coordinated by the Incident Manager and a law enforcement supervisor. A medical disaster may require National Guard or military security.

Key points for logistics systems are:

1. Determine what supplies are needed in a logistics plan.
2. Coordinate with the designated emergency management agency.
3. Identify and train supply personnel.
4. Establish disaster caches and public disaster kits.
5. Test logistics in exercises.

CHAPTER QUESTIONS/EXERCISES

1. What are the critical logistics functions in an MCI or high-impact event?
2. List and define the units in the Logistics Section.

3. Discuss the push and pull concept of logistics. Which type system (push or pull) would be most effective for your community? Why?

4. Discuss the cache method of logistics. Design an effective disaster cache suited to your locale. What supplies should be included in a public disaster kit?

5. Why is a command cache vital to an effective EMS/IMS system? What equipment/supplies should be included in a command cache?

6. What are key security issues at an MCI? What additional security issues are there in a terrorist incident?

7

COMMUNICATIONS

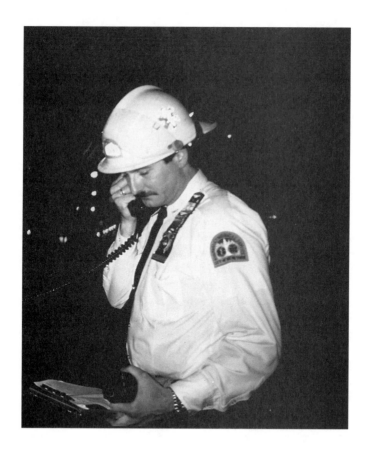

Chapter Objectives
After reading this chapter, you will be able to accomplish the following objectives:

1. Diagram and discuss the key elements in the communications model.
2. Recognize the importance of feedback in the communications process.
3. Describe the key elements in a model communications protocol.
4. Design an effective radio-failure protocol.
5. Recognize the advantages/disadvantages of basic transmission methods and hardware.
6. Define and discuss the functions of EMS communications (EMS com).
7. Define and discuss the functions of medical control.

Communications is a key component of the EMS Incident Management System. Effective communications is essential. Information must flow among all branches, sectors, and units for critical coordination to occur. There must be an effective flow of information to the Incident Manager and supporting agencies.

In the national IMS model, Communications is a support unit in the Logistics Section. This system was designed for remote deployment to wildland fires. In medical disasters, units in the EMS branch have unique communications demands. In this text, communications for EMS operations are treated as a support function to the EMS Branch. When medical communications is identified as a unit, it is called "EMS Com."

CONCEPTS VERSUS EQUIPMENT

Communications is a concept: the effective transfer of information. In disaster communications, command vehicles and radio hardware are the visual images. Hardware is essential and may have "bells and whistles." However, if the right information doesn't flow, high-tech hardware won't help. The concepts of communications must be understood for hardware to be effective.

Each unit in the IMS is a cell that exchanges information with other cells. Cells generate information ("We have two red patients"); they receive information ("We are sending ten patients to triage"); they process information ("We need ten backboards in the transportation area"). Without communications, cells become isolated, and information doesn't flow in or out. When an information vacuum exists, coordination stops and operating units lose contact and become "freelancers." At this point, there is no incident management.

Critical Factor:

The IMS does not function without effective communications.

Note that communications is information exchange, not radio traffic. Hand-held radio transmissions are the most common form of information, but information exchange is not limited to verbal methods. We can send data on computers or portable fax machines. We can transmit/receive maps, graphics, pictures, databases, and reference material between operating units. Any form of information transfer, not just verbal radio transmissions, is fair game.

Emergency radio traffic sounds chaotic. However, when the dust settles, there are several basic forms of information occurring between operational units.

1. Vehicle status—From routine incidents to disasters, vehicle availability (inservice, out of service, etc.) and vehicle location are key information. On the scene, this information is maintained by the IM and sector officers. Off the scene, this information is maintained by a dispatch center or Medical Control.

2. Unit assignments—Operational cells within the IMS (command branches, sectors, and units) receive a myriad of assignments. Assignments constantly change. As tasks are completed, new assignments are made. Incident Managers must know if an assignment is received, understood, completed, or not completed.

3. Resource consumption—Units in disasters consume resources at a horrendous rate. (See Chapter 6.) Other units are responsible for supplying the needed resources and equipment. Resource coordination is critically important. As resources are provided from farther distances (regional, state, national), communication needs grow.

4. Patient information—In medical disasters, there are continuous exchanges of data about patients. We need to know about numbers of patients, their conditions, where they are, and where they're going. This information must flow between units and outside the system to dispatch centers, Medical Control, and hospitals.

5. Emergency traffic—In any incident, things can go wrong quickly. Conditions can change that suddenly endanger patients or emergency personnel. The ability to report emergency information to all personnel and units is crucial.

THE COMMUNICATIONS MODEL

Before discussing communications networks, it is important to understand some basics about communications. If these fundamentals are ignored or misunderstood, the communications system will fail.

A message, or information exchange, can be diagrammed using the "Communications Model." Communications can be diagrammed as shown in Figure 7-1.

Each element in the Communications Model serves as a key linkage. If any element is not adequate, there is a failure to communicate. Elements are defined as:

1. Information—Information is data used to make decisions. The information must be relevant to the mission. Large amounts of raw data result in "information overload" and clutter the system. "Short and sweet" is the rule for disaster information.

2. Encoding—Encoding is changing information into an understandable format. Commonly we encode a thought into a language that is written or spoken. Thoughts and information are also encoded into pictures or graphics.

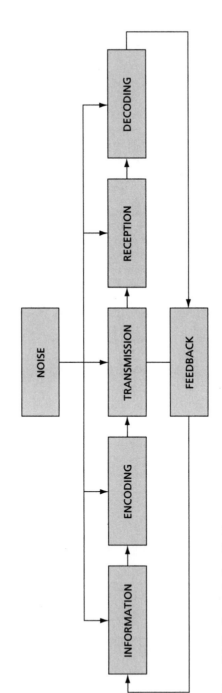

Figure 7-1 The Communications Model

3. Transmission—An encoded message has to be communicated to a receiver though a transmission. A transmission can be face-to-face, visual, or through electronic means. Historically, transmission methods have changed with technology.
4. Reception—A message has to be received. The message is processed upon reception for decoding. With electronic messages, the receiving devices must be compatible with the transmitting devices.
5. Decoding—The receiver must decode a message for understanding. Successful decoding requires familiarity with the encoding method.
6. Feedback—Feedback is acknowledgment from the receiver to the transmitter. It completes the loop.
7. Noise—Noise is interference with the communications loop. Noise may be tangible, emotional, or electronic interference. Noise is a plague to the cycle.

The Communications Model is academic, but it relates to medical disasters. The model is the basis for effective communications. When communications go bad, it's because elements in the model are missing.

COMMUNICATIONS PROTOCOL

A communications protocol is a guideline for exchanging information during emergency operations. Effective protocols must use the elements in our academic model. Let's look at the model again and translate it into a real world protocol.

First, consider the information. The information must be one of the generic forms discussed earlier (vehicle status, unit assignments, resource use, patient information, emergency traffic). Information discipline prevents overload. Transmissions should include only relevant information, and the messages should be clear and brief.

The words "emergency traffic" are key to communications protocol. "Emergency traffic" is the highest priority message. These two words give any unit free reign. Other messages stop; everyone listens.

Encoding is next. The sender has to consider the receiver's decoding ability. The most effective form of encoding is plain language. Radio codes (10 codes, Q signals, etc.) are too hard to decode. When the fire ICS was developed in the 1970s, one of the first suggestions was to remove radio codes so that diverse agencies could understand each other. STOP USING RADIO CODES. (How's that for subtlety?) Use common terminology in the IMS and plain language.

Critical Factor:

OMIT RADIO CODES; use IMS terminology and plain language.

Encoding is followed by transmission, which will be discussed in the next section. Reception and transmission are closely linked. The receiver must have compatible equipment to receive a transmission.

The common cause of reception problems is multiple agencies with different radio frequencies. The U.S. Forest Service solved this problem with radio caches. Reporting agencies leave their personal radios, and are issued a radio from the cache. Another solution is to leave an agency representative at the command post. A message is received by the IM, handed off to the agency representative, and retransmitted. This is done frequently when working with law enforcement agencies. Networks will be discussed again in a subsequent section.

Feedback is the most important element of communications. Feedback is information from the receiver back to the transmitter. Without feedback, a sender does not know if the message was received and understood.

Critical Factor:

Feedback is the most critical loop in communications.

Feedback can be positive or negative. Positive feedback means the message was received and understood. Negative feedback means it is not understood. Negative feedback sounds like:

- "I don't understand."
- "Say again."
- "I can't do it."
- "I won't do it."
- "Get a life!"

A receiving unit should identify itself and briefly restate the message. "That's a big 10-4 good buddy" is not feedback. "Transport received" is not feedback. "Transport received, you're sending three red patients" is good feedback. Air traffic control communications are examples of good feedback. When an aircraft is given instructions, the pilot always responds with the aircraft/flight number, and a repeat of the information.

If feedback is not received, the sender must assume the message was not received. The sender should try again or choose a different transmission method. It cannot be overstated; feedback is the only way to assure that communication is taking place.

Noise interferes with other elements. Tangible noise is the usual noise heard at any medical emergency. Diesels are running, people are talking (or screaming), and tools are operating. Radio transmissions may be overlapping, fragmented, full of static, or low in volume. This tangible noise interferes with message understanding.

A factor affecting a listener's physical/mental condition is intangible noise. Examples of intangible noise are stress and fatigue.

Noise can be controlled, but not eliminated. Technology can reduce tangible noise through, for example, placing managers in a communications vehicle or using noise reduction headsets. Changing transmission methods may also help. This includes face-to-face contact, laptop computers, or cellular phones. Intangible noise is harder to control. If people are tired or "stressed out," face-to-face contact is reassuring. Ultimately, they'll need a rest/rehabilitation period.

Noise problems demonstrate the importance of feedback (there's that word again). Since noise (tangible/intangible) cannot be eliminated, feedback means noise corrupted information will eventually get through. When it's noisy, numerous attempts may be needed to get positive feedback.

TRANSMISSIONS

Daily technology gives us new ways to transmit messages. Each method has good and bad features. It is important to have multiple transmission tools for two reasons:

1. Select the best form of transmission depending on the message.
2. Have alternative systems for backups.

An in-depth venture into communication technology would require volumes. In this section, we will look at an outline of basic transmission methods.

1. Public Safety Radio Network
   Advantages—Common; portable; simple; user friendly.
   Disadvantages—Very susceptible to tangible noise; frequencies not always compatible; overloads under high traffic demand; antennas susceptible to natural disaster damage; feedback only if users are highly trained.
2. Telephones (landline and cellular)
   Advantages—Portable due to cellular; most common system in the civilian community; easy to use and inexpensive; easy to solicit feedback; data capable at slow speeds.
   Disadvantages—Not all agencies have cellular; each receiver has a separate number; not effective for coordinating large numbers of units; vulnerable to natural disaster damage; can be "busied out" by disasters or high-impact events.
3. Portable Fax
   Advantages—Offers hard copy; excellent for lists, records, or large data; graphics capable.
   Disadvantages—Special equipment required; need separate transmission system (usually telephone, cellular, or RF); feedback requires other transmission.
4. Portable Computers
   Advantages—Excellent for high-speed data; automatic feedback (electronic handshake pulses).
   Disadvantages—High-tech equipment and highly trained users; expensive; requires network such as telephone, cellular, RF.

5. Runners

Advantages—Simple and low technology; backup for failed technology; feedback by face-to-face contact.

Disadvantages—Personnel intensive; low speed and short distances.

What system is the best? The answer is all of them. In most incidents, there are combinations. Examples:

1. When someone fails to answer, you send a runner. (Someone runs to a unit and says, "Why aren't you answering your radio?")
2. You use a cellular line from the IM to the communication center. If it fails (or is busy), you go back to the handheld. When the battery dies, commandeer the nearest pay phone. (Rule: The nearest phones are always vandalized.)
3. Try sending data using the new portable fax (or computer system) that was bought with a grant windfall. It worked in a drill, but won't work now; back to the handheld radio.
4. Someone always leaves his or her hand held in the station during the "big one" and must use the vehicle radio or steal another radio.

A summary of transmissions basics are:

- Use the system to suit the needs of the incident.
- Use low-tech backups when high-tech systems fail.
- Don't trust any system that has limited feedback.

COMMUNICATION PATHWAYS

In the IMS, only vehicles are identified by radio numbers. Command, sections, branches, sectors, and units are identified by their functions. Commander 403 may be assigned to triage. In a radio transmission, the expression "403" may not have any meaning to other units. The term "triage" is understood by all units. "Rescue 11 to 402" has no meaning to outside agencies. When the message is changed to "Treatment Red to Medical Sector," the functions of both elements are understood. When vehicles are identified, the agency name should precede the vehicle number. Examples include "Okaloosa Rescue 8" and "Ocean City Engine 1." This helps identify units with the same numbers or mutual aid units.

Paths can be reduced by using multiple channels or different transmission technology. Units in the Treatment Sector may use tactical channel (TAC) 1, with units in the Transportation Sector using (TAC) 2. If TAC channels are available, they can reduce frequency overload. An example of transmission modes is cellular lines between the Incident Manager and the dispatch center. This traffic pathway uses a cellular channel instead of loading an RF channel.

Establishing specific communication pathways reinforces the principle of chain of command (Chapter 1). Units assigned to specific sections, branches, or sectors talk only to their respective managers. (Emergency traffic is an exception.) A unit in Sector A does not routinely talk to Sector B or to the Branch Director. Cross traffic, bypassing the command chain, adds confusing communications chaos (an alliteration.) It excludes the assigned sector leader from the information flow.

Restricting communication does not mean units in a sector cannot talk to each other. This dilemma can be resolved by the following protocol: Direct traffic between units in a sector is permissible for exchanging direct tactical information not involving the manager.

An example, "Rescue 1 to Rescue 2; we have two backboards for you," is appropriate traffic.

SINGLE POINT OF CONTACT

The concept of a single point of contact (POC) is closely linked to the reduction of communication pathways. The POC is an individual responsible for receiving information within an agency or group of agencies. The POC is usually a section chief, branch director, or sector officer or unit leader, or an agency representative from an outside agency. The POC is important for agencies not familiar with disaster operations. Such agencies lack the "chain of command" type of organization prevalent in public safety agencies.

For the POC to be effective, critical rules must be observed:

1. The POC must monitor all communications to ensure reception of vital information.
2. The POC must pass information to all personnel and units represented by the POC.
3. The POC must "feedback" information from his/her area of responsibility to the appropriate level in the IMS.

The POC from an outside agency does not have to be a manager/decision maker. The POC has to be an information relay to the decision makers.

An example of the need for a POC is in a natural disaster where public works units from local agencies are serving as assisting agencies. Communications with each of these agencies or units will be confusing and will overload assisting agencies. There may be incompatible radio channels. If a POC is selected and issued the proper radio, there will now be a single communication contact from the IMS to the assisting units.

MODEL COMMUNICATIONS PROTOCOL

By summarizing the principles discussed, the following protocol can serve as a guide for a local model:

1. Communicate information, not data.
2. Information should be in the general categories of
   a. Vehicle status
   b. Unit assignments
   c. Resource consumption
   d. Patient information
   e. Emergency traffic

3. Replace radio codes with plain language.
4. Combat noise. Keep high level managers in a quiet area. Use alternative transmission methods in high noise areas.
5. Recognize that intangible noise (stress) inhibits communications.
6. Use multiple forms of transmission.
7. Have low-technology to back up high-technology failures.
8. Incorporate feedback in all communications procedures. Without feedback, assume the message didn't get through.
9. Reduce communications paths to eliminate overload and confusion.
10. EMERGENCY TRAFFIC HAS PRIORITY. It always gets through.
11. Identify units by their IMS function instead of unit numbers or titles.
12. Establish a single point of contact for outside agencies.
13. Have a radio cache.

BRIEFINGS

Face-to-face meetings are regarded as a communication tool. In an MCI, things move fast; there isn't time to have a lengthy conference.

Briefings provide the most effective feedback. Facial expressions, hand gestures, and body language communicate ideas that cannot be exchanged in other formats. Placing a hand on someone's shoulder, looking the person in the eye, and saying, "Go do it," has great impact.

Schedule briefings among key leaders in long-term operations as required. During a twelve-hour Haz Mat incident, briefings may be every two hours. During a hurricane or earthquake recovery, a morning and evening briefing will work.

Briefings should be organized observing the following guidelines:

1. Identify key managers for the meetings.
2. Include elected officials if they are present.
3. Select a briefing site. Use a building or communications van. Get away from the noise and out of the weather if possible.
4. Exclude the media; issue a media release later.
5. Take notes.
6. Keep the meeting *short and focused.*
7. Solicit candid feedback.
8. Cover the questions:
   a. Where have we been?
   b. Where are we?
   c. Where are we going?
9. Schedule additional briefings and stick to the schedule.

Everyone learns at briefings. Often, confusion is uncovered and the Incident Action Plan changes. Schedule periodic briefings; they're worth the time.

COMMUNICATION SECURITY

Traditional public safety RF systems are not secure. Many people are listening because radio scanners are cheap and plentiful. What you say can be held against you. (Codes don't provide security; the eavesdroppers know the codes.)

Determine what information is secure. This may include patient data, especially if names are used. The names of killed or injured operations personnel must be confidential. Law enforcement information, communicated openly, can jeopardize a game plan. (The bad guys can be listening.) Lastly, some forms of information need to be media secure. (The media listens too.)

When transmitting secure information, select a safe communication medium. Forget radio traffic; it's wide open. An exception is digital 800 MHz transmissions, which are somewhat more secure. (Note: Radio traffic can be scrambled, but the receiver must have the same type of scrambler.) Cellular traffic is more secure than RF, but can be monitored with scanners. Hard wire telephone lines are vulnerable, but much better than radio traffic. Computer data, transmitted by RF, cellular, or land lines provide a higher security level.

EMS COM

On routine incidents, a paramedic gives a patient report to the receiving medical facility. In an MCI or disaster, communicating detailed patient information is not practical. Detailed reports on multiple patients will overload communication channels. The treatment personnel are too busy for long conversations.

A solution in the IMS is an EMS communicator, or EMS Com. At an MCI, EMS Com works in the EMS Branch. EMS Com is the single point of contact (remember the POC concept) for patient information. (See Figure 7-2.)

EMS Com roams the incident area and receives basic patient information from each treatment team. The EMS Com report should include:

1. Number of patients
2. Condition of patients (red, yellow, or green)
3. Special information (pediatric, pregnancy, etc.)

An example of an efficient EMS Com report is, "EMS Com to Medical Control; we have four red, two yellow, one pediatric trauma alert." The objective is to transmit patient information in a brief and concise manner. (This information will lead to efficient patient transportation.)

The person selected needs only a basic medical background. The ability to understand IMS terminology and have basic communication skills are the basic requirements. The treatment unit leader can serve as Med Com if other personnel are not available.

The EMS Com concept provides a key link between treatment teams and Medical Control. EMS Com provides patient reports, without committing medical

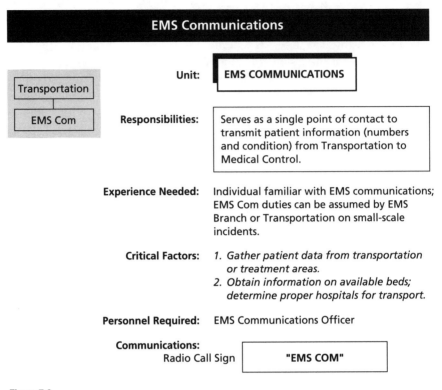

Figure 7-2

personnel to communication duties. The information supplied by EMS Com is ultimately used by Medical Control to determine transport priorities and locations.

MEDICAL CONTROL

Medical Control serves as the gatekeeper during multiple patient incidents. Medical Control is responsible for maintaining the patient receiving status for all medical facilities in the region. Medical Control, after receiving EMS Com reports, determines what patients go where. This information is communicated to Transport.

Medical Control is usually located at a dispatch center or hospital command post. During an MCI, Medical Control contacts all appropriate medical facilities to determine patient availability and maintain status of specialized facilities, such as burn units, pediatric hospitals, etc.

Medical Control, especially in dispatch centers, can serve as the catalyst that gets the system in motion in a major incident. Notification of Medical Control initiates checklists based on the severity of the problem. (Checklists are maintained for MCIs and medical disasters.) These checklists include key personnel, support agencies, all regional medical facilities, and mutual aid agencies. A notification from an Incident Manager is the trigger to initiate the Medical Control checklists. The words, "We have a mass casualty incident" can boost the emergency medical system into "after-burner" by the actions of Medical Control.

COMMUNICATIONS FAILURE PROTOCOL

In EMS, communications is an essential element that is taken for granted until it fails. Any number of factors can cause the EMS radio system to fail. Natural disasters such as earthquakes, hurricanes, floods, and tornadoes can cause the telephone system, cellular system, and radio system to simultaneously fail. Suddenly, all units are operating in a vacuum. If there is no written protocol, it's too late to instruct isolated units.

A communications failure protocol must be tailor made for each agency. Regardless of the community, a protocol must answer the following questions:

- What do units do when radios, telephones, or both fail?
- What backup hardware is available for a "quick fix?"

In a telephone system failure, internal EMS operations are not hampered. However, citizens cannot call 9-1-1. The public should be instructed to report to the nearest EMS, fire, or police station to report an incident. Immediately public instructions can be conveyed through the media.

When the EMS radio system fails, the opposite happens. EMS operations are hampered, but the public still has 9-1-1. In this case, units must be dispatched by telephone and be instructed to standby at stations or hospitals to maintain telephone contact. If units have cellular telephones, the dispatch problem is partially solved. (Many members have personal cellular telephones and/or pagers. These numbers should be available to the dispatch center.)

When everything fails, the public and EMS alike are in a blackout. Units should be instructed to remain at their stations. Large numbers of patients may report to public safety facilities for aid. (Remember to have disaster caches.) Citizens can also report incidents remote from the reporting site. (Note: There should be a continuous public education program instructing citizens where to seek aid in a disaster.)

If a total communications failure is due to a disaster, several steps are important:

- Nonambulance vehicles (usually their managers/supervisors) must perform a damage assessment of key hospitals to determine suitability for patient reception.
- Extra members must be pre-assigned to stations to perform treatment of walk-in patients.
- Units should recon high-density areas to determine if there are mass casualties.

Back-up hardware can also be an effective solution. A disaster seldom destroys the amateur radio network. By pre-arrangement, amateur radio operators can report to designated areas and set up transceivers, antennas, and repeaters.

Satellite telephones are very effective. These units are portable and can operate anywhere on Earth. With a cost of under three thousand dollars, agencies can afford back-up satellite units at essential stations.

With the potential for an existing communications infrastructure to be rendered useless or destroyed, the EMS system and its medical director should be prepared to fall back on "standing orders" for patient care. There may be some reluctancy on the part of the medical director who must authorize the use of "standing orders," but the usefulness of this "medical privilege" cannot be overemphasized. Remember, what you are attempting to achieve is a maintenance of service when you are in the middle of a high-impact event and the bottom has dropped out (e.g., no telemetry or dispatch radio.) By getting your medical director involved in the development of this radio failure protocol from the beginning, you will foster a full understanding of the goals of the protocols while permitting the medical director to put in place safeguards to ensure proper and effective patient care in times of system crisis. Surely from an ALS perspective, having limited "standing orders" beats falling back on BLS treatment and transport for that patient in dire need of ALS.

SUMMARY

The IMS cannot function without effective communications. Each element in the IMS is a cell that exchanges information with other cells. The five forms of information that must be communicated are unit status, unit assignments, resource consumption, patient information, and emergency traffic.

All forms of information are exchanged through the communications model. Information is encoded, transmitted, received, and decoded. The receiver responds back to the transmitter by a feedback loop. Tangible and intangible noise interferes with the communication process.

A communications protocol serves as a guideline for effective procedures. Key elements in a protocol include information categories, use of plain language, multiple forms of transmission, a backup system, feedback, reduced communications paths, identity of units by function, and establishment of a single point of contact for outside agencies.

Periodic face-to-face briefings are important during long-duration operations. Briefings include key players and cover the basic questions of "Where have we been? Where are we? Where are we going?"

EMS Com is the element responsible for gathering patient information from treatment teams and relaying to Medical Control. Medical Control is a dispatch center or hospital command post that maintains the patient status of all medical facilities.

CHAPTER QUESTIONS/EXERCISES

1. Diagram the Communications Model. What is the key element in the model that ensures effective communications?
2. What types of information should be communicated during major operations?
3. What elements should be included in a communications protocol? Outline a protocol for your EMS agency.
4. What is a radio failure protocol? Write a basic radio failure protocol for your emergency response agency.
5. List and define five different forms of communications technology. What are advantages and disadvantages of each technology?
6. Discuss why radio codes should be eliminated from emergency response agencies.
7. Define and discuss the duties of EMS Com.
8. What are the responsibilities of Medical Control?

8

THE CHEMICAL ENVIRONMENT

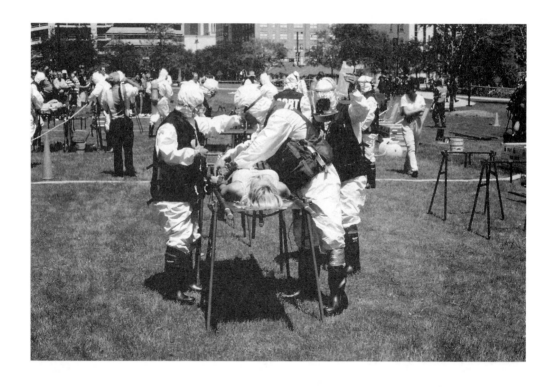

Chapter Objectives
After reading this chapter, you will be able to accomplish the following objectives:

1. Understand the principle of mechanism of injury and how it relates to hazardous chemical exposure.
2. List and discuss the function of the decon unit, including the unit's relationship to triage.
3. Describe the principles of effective decontamination.
4. List and discuss the supplies and equipment needed in a decon kit.
5. Understand the concept of a Technical Advisor and how it relates to Haz Mat operations.
6. Discuss reference materials and sources of reference information for Haz Mat incidents.
7. Discuss the requirements of a hospital decon protocol.
8. Discuss the functions of a medical unit in the hazardous materials ICS.
9. Recognize the importance of detection and mass decontamination in a chemical-biological terrorism incident.

THE CHEMICAL ENVIRONMENT

We live in a chemical society. Although exact numbers are debatable, chemical experts agree there are over one hundred thousand hazardous materials in our society. Chemicals are also effective terrorist weapons. These materials can be solids, liquids, or gases. They produce acute trauma such as radiation burns, pulmonary edema, respiratory arrest, explosion injuries, and neurological damage. Chronic effects include gradual organ dysfunction, infertility, birth defects, and cancer.

Chemicals that produce harmful vapors can spread over a large area. With railroad or maritime quantities, or a chemical-biological attack, there is potential for hundreds of patients.

An effective management system anticipates the need for decontaminating and treating chemically exposed patients. Medical treatment protocols for chemical emergencies change as our knowledge of toxicology progresses. Exact protocols will not be discussed. However, reference sources will be covered in a later section.

MECHANISM OF INJURY

A key concept in emergency medical care is mechanism of injury. Mechanism of injury is a sudden intense energy that is transmitted to the body and causes trauma. The chest hitting the steering wheel in an MVA, a bullet entering the body, or the sudden stop after a fall are all mechanisms of injury. In each case, the mechanism lasts a second or less and is depleted by the time first responders arrive.

Normal mechanism of injury concepts do not apply with hazardous materials exposure or chemical weapons. If the patient is touching, ingesting, or breathing the material, the mechanism of injury persists. If EMS responders become exposed to the chemical source, they will be affected by the mechanism of injury. If the patient is not decontaminated, the situation gets worse, because transporting the patient brings the mechanism of injury to the hospital. Chemical fumes can be circulated in the hospital air conditioning system and can injure medical personnel and patients.

Critical Factor:

In chemical exposures, the mechanism of injury can last for an extended period and expose treatment personnel and patients to chemical trauma.

The objective, in any hazardous materials or terrorist chemical attack incident, is to remove the mechanism of injury quickly. Remember, the mechanism affects everyone, including John Wayne type rescuers.

CASE HISTORIES

Several recent incidents demonstrate the seriousness of chemical injuries in disasters and the danger of a lingering mechanism of injury.

CASE 1: A helicopter air ambulance crew assisted in extrication operations at a vehicle rollover. The truck was not placarded and had no shipping papers. Its cargo was organic pesticides. The helicopter crew showed minor signs of chemical exposure. After several days, exposure symptoms worsened. It was discovered that the leather flight boots were contaminated. The mechanism of injury had been removed from the patients, but stayed with the rescuers.

CASE 2: Two laborers were exposed to a chlorine leak. They were treated on the scene for respiratory exposure and transported to the hospital in their work clothes. They were examined and released, only to return to the scene still reeking of chlorine. The injury mechanism left the scene and came back.

CASE 3: An explosion and fire in an office complex resulted in several patients being transported. ER personnel noted that the patients smelled like chemicals, and their hair was melting. Doctors and nurses began to cough. Other staff members and patients smelled chemical fumes coming from air conditioning ducts. The ER had to be evacuated and decontaminated by a fire department hazardous materials team. It was discovered that patients had been exposed to corrosive chemicals used in photocopying. In this case, the mechanism of injury visited the hospital and decided to roam around.

CASE 4: In Tokyo, Japan, a fanatical religious group intentionally released Sarin (nerve gas) in the subway system. There were multiple casualties. There were additional casualties to paramedics, firefighters, and police officers due to chemical exposure.

In each case, the Incident Management System failed to properly respond to the chemical problem. In the EMS Incident Management System, a decontamination (decon) unit must be established whenever chemical or hazardous materials exposure is confirmed or suspected. (See Figure 8-1.)

THE DECON UNIT

When hazardous materials are present at an emergency incident or disaster, patients must be decontaminated before or during medical treatment. In the EMS Incident Management System, a decon unit is a team assigned to decontaminate chemically exposed patients. Contaminated patients are usually discovered during triage. The patients must be removed from the source of the exposure and decontaminated, before routing to a treatment area in order to protect rescuers and expedite patient care.

The decon unit is supervised by the Haz Mat Branch Director. If patients are in a known chemical hot zone, they are removed by rescuers and pass through a

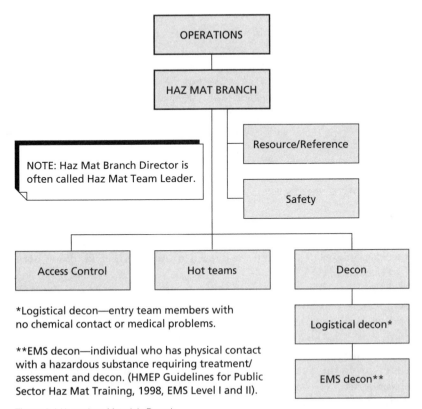

*Logistical decon—entry team members with no chemical contact or medical problems.

**EMS decon—individual who has physical contact with a hazardous substance requiring treatment/ assessment and decon. (HMEP Guidelines for Public Sector Haz Mat Training, 1998, EMS Level I and II).

Figure 8-1 Hazardous Materials Branch

decontamination corridor operated by the decon unit. These patients are routed through the EMS Branch for triage, treatment, and transport.

Many disasters are not actual chemical incidents, but involve large numbers of chemically exposed patients. Examples are natural disasters and transportation accidents. Most of the victims are trauma patients, mixed with chemically contaminated patients. In these situations, victims are dispersed over a wide area. Contamination is discovered by EMS teams during triage. The decon unit has to be mobile and decontaminate patients in place, or move them to a decon area. Affected patients must be decontaminated before they are moved to a treatment area. Remember, the chemical mechanism of injury will continually harm the patient, rescuers, EMS personnel, and other patients.

Critical Factor:

Chemically contaminated patients must be decontaminated before medical treatment.

The decon unit/sector should be staffed by appropriately trained and equipped rescuers. The proper personal protection equipment (PPE) is essential when hazards are present, as is having the experience and knowledge to properly execute decisions relative to the selection of the type of PPE. No decision that the decon unit leader will make is more important than the determination of level of protection for both the respiratory protection or suit selection. There is a real big difference in the level of protection afforded between, let's say, a self-contained breathing apparatus and an air purifying respirator. The personnel assigned to perform decon duties need to have not only a high level of medical training, but also a high skill level in Haz Mat operations.

PRINCIPLES OF DECONTAMINATION

In the 1980s, decontamination procedures were complex. There were five decon solutions (A to E) recommended, depending on the chemical. Some of the solutions were weak acids or alkali agents, designed to neutralize acid/base chemicals and could cause harm.

Today, the decontamination process is simplified. The patient, after clothing removal, is washed with water or a light detergent, or wiped with dry cloths, depending on the chemical. Warning: *Water is suitable for most chemicals, but may be harmful in some cases; use an adequate reference source to determine the decon protocol.*

The basic principles of decon are not "rocket scientist" concepts. Removing the patient from the hot zone and removing the patient's clothing are the basics. (If possible, bag the clothing and leave it in the hot zone for disposal. Jewelry and personal effects can be separately bagged for reclaiming.)

The principles of patient decon are summarized as:

1. Move the patient away from further exposure.
2. Remove the patient's clothing and jewelry.
3. Wash the patient, or use dry wiping for water reactive materials.

Remember the decon saying is: "Move 'em, strip 'em, and clean 'em."

DECON EQUIPMENT

Basic equipment for decontamination includes the following categories:

1. Personal Protective Equipment (PPE)
2. Washing equipment
3. Containment equipment

PPE is necessary to protect the decon unit. Respiratory equipment and protective suits and gloves are required. Reference materials will indicate minimum suit requirements appropriate for a given chemical. In many cases, a Tyvek disposable suit (Saranex coated), with a hood and booties, will be adequate. Firefighting turnout gear or work uniforms will absorb chemicals, become permanently contaminated, and serve as a mechanism of injury.

Washing equipment consists of soft bristle brushes (dish mops will work), sponges, a soft detergent, towels, and water.

Containment equipment prevents chemical runoff from causing environmental damage. This consists of a roll of plastic, or a vinyl fire salvage cover, and an inexpensive children's inflatable pool. Water that runs off the patient is contained by the pool or plastic sheeting. A disposal bag is used to store contaminated clothing or clean-up equipment.

Emergency operations can result in the uniforms of EMS personnel being contaminated. Shoes are famous for absorbing liquid chemicals; all contaminated clothing must be immediately removed and bagged. EMS units should carry inexpensive disposable coveralls that can be donned after uniform removal. This provides your members with a garment until they return to the station.

MASS DECONTAMINATION

With the advent of chemical-biological terrorism, there is a possibility that hundreds of patients must be decontaminated. The military considers mass decon of trained soldiers a major problem. With civilian children and the elderly, the problem is monumental.

Traditional decon, utilizing inflatable pools, is not practical. Fixed spray systems, with lines of ambulatory patients, are a possible solution. The patients must be de-clothed before the decon process. After decon, disposable suits (Tyvek for example) will be needed for privacy and environmental exposure.

Non-ambulatory patients present a more serious problem. Each patient needs individual attention; contaminated litters will not be able to enter the clean area, but must be rotated back into the hot zone. This means litter changes at the clean end of the decon corridor.

A national protocol for civilian mass decontamination is not available at the time of publication of this text. However, such protocols are being drafted, with assistance from military experts.

TECHNICAL ADVISOR

The Technical Advisor, in the IMS model, is any individual with specialized expertise. The Technical Advisor is an important component in the IMS toolbox when hazardous materials or military chemicals are involved. Toxicologists, military specialists, and industrial hygienists can provide expert advice on decontamination and treatment procedures. A Poison Control Center is another source of technical advice, especially in the absence of local expertise. Since most physicians do not have the in-depth toxicology background necessary to give adequate support, it is important to include a Technical Advisor in disaster pre-planning.

REFERENCE MATERIALS

With over one hundred thousand known hazardous chemicals, it is impossible to memorize even a fraction of them. One of the most important medical tools is chemical reference books.

The first step in using reference materials is to identify the chemical. Correct spelling is important, as one incorrect letter can change the name of a chemical to a different substance. If the name of the chemical cannot be obtained, try to determine the general classification from a shipping label. General classifications are explosives, combustible liquids, corrosive materials, flammable liquids, flammable gases, nonflammable gases, flammable solids, organic peroxides, oxidizers, poisons, etiologic agents, and radioactive materials.

EMS providers need, as a minimum, the *DOT North American Emergency Response Guide*. The book is written in plain language and serves as a quick reference source. The guide describes BLS treatment for the chemicals listed. ALS units need reference books with ALS procedures and decon protocols.

The local hazardous materials team needs extensive reference materials. In the hazardous materials IMS, there is a Resource/Reference Officer (Figure 8-1). This position is responsible for obtaining all possible data on given chemicals. The

Resource/Reference Officer may also access on-line computer databases, Material Safety Data Sheets (MSDS), and faxed information by cellular telephone.

Another important reference source is CHEMTREC. This is a chemical information center established as public service by the Chemical Manufacturers Association. CHEMTREC is accessible 24 hours a day at 800-424-9300.

HOSPITAL DECONTAMINATION

Joint accreditation standards require that hospital emergency departments have a plan for chemically contaminated patients. Contaminated patients are an infrequent hospital occurrence and present an unpleasant surprise to the ED staff. Hospitals cannot assume the EMS system will deliver a clean patient. Patients also arrive by private vehicle, making the hospital the first step in the decon process, instead of the last. A hospital needs a decontamination plan that specifies which personnel perform decon operations, define a decon area, and list decon procedures and equipment.

PERSONAL PROTECTIVE EQUIPMENT AND TRAINING

Hospital emergency department personnel may be called upon to perform patient care and decontamination within the hospital. These personnel may be exposed to a significant risk of secondary contamination from their patients. In addition, these personnel may be called upon to assist prehospital personnel requiring technical assistance in patient decontamination.

Consistent with the demands of rendering care to a contaminated patient, hospital and ED administrators must review the legislative and professional mandates for training and equipping staff members. (Refer to JCAHO and HMTUSA guidelines.) "At a minimum, hospital personnel must be able to analyze the situation, assess patient conditions and problems, take the necessary steps to assure medical provider safety, attempt identificaiton of the offending chemical substance, and initiate the decontamination and medical care process." (HMTUSA 1997 Guideline For Public Sector Hazardous Materials Training-Hospital Personnel.)

An important element in a hospital decon protocol is the identification of an emergency decontamination area. This area should be an outside location, separate from return air intakes to the hospital air conditioning/ventilation system. A water spigot should be accessible for washdown purposes. A loading dock (if it is close to the ED), or a covered entrance-way, provides a good decon area. Many hospitals are designing state-of-the-art decon facilities, and building them into new ERs. Plastic sheeting and/or a water recovery pool prevents floor or ground contamination. It is important to cover floor drains to isolate the drainage system from chemical runoff. A decon area exposes a patient to the weather and does not provide privacy. However, outside decon is necessary in extreme cases to avoid the dire consequences of chemical liquids or vapors penetrating treatment rooms or entering the air conditioning system.

All decon materials can be kept in a kit and stored near the decontamination area. The kit is inexpensive and includes:

1. A decon checklist
2. A copy of the hospital decontamination protocol
3. Reference materials and telephone numbers
4. Disposable coveralls and chemical gloves
5. Washing materials, decon solution, and towels
6. Plastic sheeting, inflatable pools, and collection/containment equipment, if required
7. Garden hose, spray nozzle, and water source

HAZARDOUS MATERIALS TEAM SUPPORT

An EMS unit is an important team in the hazardous materials team's Incident Management System (Figure 8-1). The EMS unit coordinates with the Decontamination Officer and Safety Officer, and is commanded by the Haz Mat team leader (NOTE: The EMS unit is not assigned to an EMS Branch, but works with the Fire/Rescue Branch).

The primary function of the EMS unit is to conduct medical surveillance of hazardous materials team members before entry and after exiting the decontamination area. The medical unit is positioned near the cold (clean) side of the decontamination corridor. The most common medical problems of Haz Mat team members are fatigue and heat stress from working in chemical suits. Members with high BP or heart rates, or high body temperatures, cannot report to a staging area for re-suiting. Chemical exposure or trauma can occur to a Haz Mat team, but it is not common.

The key functions of the EMS unit supporting a hazardous materials team are:

1. The EMS unit is a component of the Haz Mat team IMS and assigned to the Haz Mat team leader.
2. The EMS unit coordinates with the Haz Mat Safety Officer and decon unit.
3. The EMS unit is vulnerable to chemical injury and must remain in the "cold zone."
4. The EMS unit's mission is to evaluate and/or treat team members or victims after decontamination.
5. The EMS unit may utilize the Resource/Reference Officer for chemical information.

SUMMARY

Hazardous materials exposures and chemical terrorism present an unusual mechanism of injury. This mechanism can continue to expose a patient and/or harm medical personnel. If a patient is not decontaminated, the hospital emergency department and other patients can be exposed.

Patients exposed to hazardous materials must be decontaminated before the triage. The decon unit is an element in the IMS and is assigned decon responsibilities. The decon unit is staffed by rescuers with breathing apparatus and appropriate personal protective equipment (PPE). The decon unit is responsible for removing patients from the chemical hot zone and decontaminating the patient. The patient is then routed to the triage unit.

The principles of patient decontamination are the removal of contaminated clothing and shoes, and rinsing/washing chemicals from the patient's hair and skin. Water reactive chemicals must be removed by dry towels. Decontamination equipment includes washing supplies and containment material to confine runoff.

A Technical Advisor is any individual with specialized expertise. Industrial hygienists, military specialists, and toxicologists are technical experts who can assist physicians in providing treatment advice for chemical injuries. Reference materials that contain ALS treatment protocols and decontamination procedures are sources of information. Computer databases, Material Safety Data Sheets, military manuals, and CHEMTREC provide additional assistance.

Hospitals are required to have a procedure for on-site chemical decontamination. Hospital personnel, usually emergency department staff, need PPE, washing materials, containment material, and reference sources. These supplies are carried in a decon kit. A decon area, separate from the building's air conditioning system, must be established.

An EMS unit provides support to the hazardous materials ICS. The EMS unit is managed by the Haz Mat team leader, and coordinates with the Safety Officer and decon unit. The EMS unit evaluates the Haz Mat team members or patients after they exit the decon corridor. The tasks and knowledge required of a Haz Mat team member exceed that of a basic emergency responder. The intent of this chapter is to allow the basic responder to develop a fundamental understanding of the complexities involved with a hazardous materials emergency response. A variety of standards exist that the responder or organization must consult regarding training and operations. Some such standards are 29 CFR 1910.120, EPA 311, NFPA 471, 472, and 473, and the Hazardous Materials Uniform Transportation Safety Act's *Guidelines for Public Sector Hazardous Materials Training,* to name a few. The reader is strongly encouraged to consult these and other guidelines and to successfully complete a certified hazardous material training program prior to executing hazardous materials response actions. Successful completion of the program exceeds the responders' current sanctioned certification level.

CHAPTER QUESTIONS/EXERCISES

1. What is "mechanism of injury"? Why is the chemical mechanism of injury unique compared to trauma?
2. At the next training meeting, discuss several local case histories where chemical contamination was a factor. What decon procedures were used? What protocols or equipment are needed to control future chemical exposure incidents?
3. What is the decon unit? Diagram the decon unit in the IMS.

4. What are the principles of decontamination?
5. What equipment, supplies, and materials should be carried in a decon kit?
6. What is a Technical Advisor? How does this position relate to hazardous materials? What Technical Advisors are in the local and regional area?
7. What reference materials should be available to the decon unit? What are other sources of chemical reference material?
8. What are the essential steps in a hospital decon protocol? What materials should be contained in the hospital decon kit?
9. What is the function of the EMS unit in the support of an operating hazardous materials team?

9

COMMUNITY THREAT ASSESSMENT

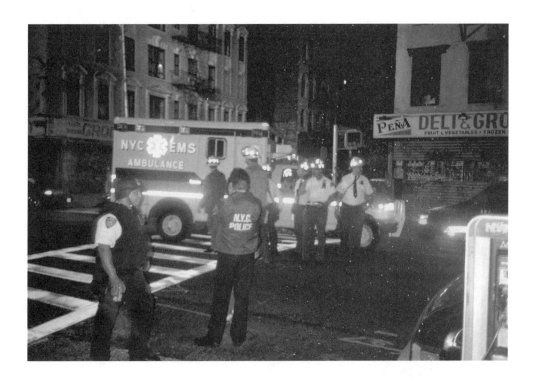

Chapter Objectives

After reading this chapter, you will be able to accomplish the following objectives:

1. Analyze the potential for natural and technological disasters in the region.
2. Understand the importance of a Disaster Committee and how it can be organized.
3. Describe the concept of Emergency Support Functions (ESF).
4. Integrate ESFs into the Incident Management System (IMS).
5. List the steps in developing a Disaster Plan.
6. Use the ESF concept and the IMS model for major event planning.
7. Discuss common problems that occur in most disaster incidents.

COMMUNITY THREAT ASSESSMENT

In previous chapters, we examined the relationship of operations, logistics, and communications. In a large MCI, or a medical disaster, a successful outcome depends on dozens of agencies. Many of these agencies do not normally work together. If they do not meet, plan, and train, they will not effectively coordinate on the "big one." The emergency medical community cannot support a major incident without the full resources of other organizations.

The local area or region needs a Disaster Committee and a Community Disaster Plan. The networking of a Disaster Committee, and a resultant Disaster Plan, can ensure that the support elements in IMS coordinate effectively.

THE DISASTER COMMITTEE

A vehicle for bringing all of the community disaster players together is a local/regional Disaster Committee. A Disaster Committee can take a variety of forms in communities such as Emergency Control Board, local Emergency Planning Committee, etc. Any person, agency, or organization that has a logistical, planning, or operational role in emergency operations should be included.

The functions of the Disaster Committee should include:

1. Establish a forum for threat/risk assessment.
2. Serve as a vehicle for emergency response planning.
3. Establish disaster exercises.
4. Evaluate overall disaster plans.
5. Mediate disputes between response agencies.
6. Conduct post-incident analysis.
7. Serve as a conduit for public/private partnerships.
8. Maintain a database of emergency response resources.

It is obvious that response agencies belong on a disaster committee. But support agencies may not be aware of their roles. Some law enforcement agencies have to be urged to join disaster planning efforts. The local power company, council on aging, transportation authority, or the amateur radio club may not appreciate its value to the response agencies.

COMMUNITY THREAT/RISK POTENTIAL

Every locale in the world is vulnerable to numerous potential hazards. There are case histories that serve as constant reminders. California has earthquakes, the Midwest has tornado alley, and Florida has hurricanes. However, other threats, waiting to happen, are not readily apparent.

At the first meeting of the new Disaster Committee, conduct a local threat assessment. Use the Community Threat Assessment form (Figure 9-1). The disasters

---

SCORE: H – High risk
         M – Moderate risk
         L – Low risk
         O – No risk

1. Nuclear attack	___	13. Winter storm	___
2. Terrorism	___	14. Hurricane	___
3. Civil disorder	___	15. Tornado	___
4. Criminal disorder	___	16. Flood	___
5. Earthquake	___	17. Wildfire	___
6. Tidal wave	___	18. Urban fire	___
7. Volcano	___	19. Transportation	___
8. Avalanche	___	20. Haz Mat (trans.)	___
9. Landslide	___	21. Haz Mat (facility)	___
10. Dam failure	___	22. Radiological (trans.)	___
11. Power failure	___	23. Radiological (facility)	___
12. Disease	___	24. Subsidence (sinkholes)	___

TOTAL HIGH ___
TOTAL MOD ___
TOTAL LOW ___

Figure 9-1 Community Threat Assessment

are divided into two categories, technological and natural. Each potential disaster is rated as:

1. No risk—no previous history; no likely chance of occurrence. (Example: avalanche in Miami)
2. Low risk—very limited history; possible but not likely. (Example: radiological transportation accident in a rural area)
3. Moderate risk—historical likelihood; moderate frequency and/or moderate severity. (Example: airplane crash in a suburban area)
4. High risk—frequent history; high potential for severe incident. (Example: wildfires in California, rural-urban interface areas).

NOTE: History can change threat assessments. There was a time when Oklahoma City would have been rated as a low risk for terrorism.

Answers on the Community Threat Assessment form are subjective. If the values scored by local "experts" are compared, patterns will emerge. The total scores aren't important; identification of potential threats are what we're looking for.

A community threat analysis directs planning efforts for special problems. If a large potential for chemical incidents is identified, plans are made to establish a hazardous materials team and/or identify mutual aid resources and logistics needs. If there is an avalanche problem, special rescue teams are equipped and trained to respond.

The problems identified in the disaster potential survey provide a strong argument for an Incident Management System (IMS). It is not feasible to have a separate plan for each type of incident. It is a proven concept that the IMS is effective on any type of problem, especially if the support needs and special teams are identified.

TERRORISM THREAT ASSESSMENT

The World Trade Center bombing, the Oklahoma City tragedy, and the Atlanta bombings have jolted America into an awakening; terrorism is here. The reasons are numerous and varied and beyond the scope of this text. The Sarin gas attack in the Tokyo subway system marked the beginning of a new and insidious form of urban terror; the chemical-biological threat is a reality.

Federal threat assessments indicate that local communities are vulnerable. A terrorist attack with weapons of mass destruction is a viable supposition. In the old days, a local/regional EMS Disaster Plan only included an analysis of natural and technological hazards. The need for a terrorism threat assessment is a twenty-first century reality. Any community is a possibility. Key threat issues include:

1. High crowd areas—sporting events, concerts, festivals, religious services.
2. Transportation—airports, underground trains, tunnels, ships.
3. Buildings—public safety, federal, schools, religious, computer centers.
4. Utilities—water, power stations, gas, telephone.
5. Special events—celebrities, national/international political figures.
6. Hazardous materials storage areas.

If possible, EMS agencies should have access to non-classified intelligence information from local and federal law enforcement sources. Security concerns may result in only limited data at the local level, but it's worth a try.

EMERGENCY SUPPORT FUNCTIONS

In the 1980s the Federal Government drafted the Federal Response Plan (FRP). The FRP identified twelve Emergency Support Functions (ESF). Each ESF had a support, planning, or operational function. A lead agency was identified, along with support agencies. For example, the medical function is ESF 8, Health and Medical. The lead agency is the Department of Health and Human Services. The main response component is the U.S. Public Health Service, through the National Disaster Medical System. The support agencies are the Military Medical Commands in the Department of Defense.

Each Secretary (Cabinet level) signed the FRP. Many of the participating agencies were not familiar with their roles, making the FRP essentially a "paper" plan. This changed dramatically in 1992 with Hurricane Andrew. The Federal Government implemented the FRP on a major scale. Midlevel department heads and military commanders quickly learned about the FRP. After Andrew, the Emergency Support Functions (ESF) were battle tested and fared well.

The State of Florida adopted the twelve original ESFs, and added four more (See Figure 9-2). This program was implemented by the Division of Emergency Management. At the county level, emergency management adopted the same ESFs and identified lead agencies, with related support organizations.

When examining the list of ESFs, emergency agencies are easily identified (Example: ESF 4 (Firefighting) is assigned to Fire/Rescue agencies.) Nonresponse ESF agencies are not so readily identified. They include transportation, communications, mass care, resource support, food and water, and volunteers.

The list of local agencies relating to each ESF may or may not apply to your local area. One of the first steps for your new Disaster Committee will be to identify a lead agency and several secondary agencies for each ESF. The Emergency Management Director should take the lead in this effort. When it's done, the Director will have 90% of his/her Disaster Plan completed.

Consider Food and Water, ESF 11, in a hypothetical community. The Salvation Army has a disaster van that is used as a mobile kitchen. The American Red Cross has a similar unit; either agency could be assigned the lead. Both agencies also have ESF 11 counterparts at the state and federal levels.

In this example, further discussion and research reveals other secondary ESF 11 agencies. The county agricultural agent has access to state and federal food surplus. The local ecumenical council has a list of volunteer religious organizations that operate portable kitchens. Private, fast-food franchises also provide free food as a community service during disasters. A local milk company can haul potable water with its stainless steel tank trucks.

Figure 9-2 ESF Chart

ESF	STATE AGENCY	LOCAL AGENCIES
1. Transportation	Dept. of Transportation	Transit Authority, School Board, Council on Aging
2. Communications	Dept. of Management Services	Telephone Company, Emergency Management, Amateur Radio
3. Public Works	Dept. of Transportation	County and Local Public Works, Construction Contractors
4. Firefighting	Dept. of Insurance	Fire/Rescue Dept., Div. of Forestry
5. Information and Planning	Dept. of Community Affairs	Emergency Management, Planning Dept.
6. Mass Care	American Red Cross	American Red Cross, School Board
7. Resource Support	Dept. of Management Services	Purchasing Dept.
8. Health and Medical	Dept. of Health	Emergency Medical Services, Private Health Agencies, Public Health
9. Search and Rescue	Dept. of Insurance	Fire/Rescue, Volunteer Search Teams, Civil Air Patrol
10. Hazardous Materials	Dept. of Environmental Protection	Emergency Management, Fire/Rescue
11. Food and Water	Dept. of Agriculture and Consumer Affairs	Salvation Army, Agricultural Agent, Red Cross, Water Dept.
12. Energy	Public Service Commission	Power Company, Gas District, Public Works
13. Military Support	Dept. of Military Affairs	Emergency Management
14. Public Information	Dept. of Community Affairs	Emergency Management, County and Local PIO
15. Volunteers and Donations	Dept. of Community Affairs	Emergency Management, United Way, Religious Organizations
16. Law Enforcement	Dept. of Law Enforcement	Sheriff's Dept., Local Police

Note: State agencies are from the State of Florida; some areas have added animal control as an ESF 17

With research, you can discover more agencies in the community that provide ESF 11 services. When this process is repeated with all sixteen ESFs, a comprehensive list is created. More importantly, this confirmation of lead agencies and secondary agencies is the basis for a Community Disaster Plan.

The State of Florida has written extensive manuals for each ESF. These manuals suggest appropriate agencies and standard operating procedures. They also present a suggested chain of command and information flow within each ESF. This information saves time during a local organizing effort. FEMA, along with state and local emergency management offices, are sources of reference materials and expertise.

After identifying participating agencies, the Disaster Committee should meet with each agency's representative. A Memorandum of Understanding (MOU) between the agency and local emergency management should be developed. A simple MOU will suffice. Lawyers may not agree, but a complicated legal agreement is not necessary. An MOU formalizes the relationship between the various agencies in the Incident Management System and clarifies the agency's responsibility.

INCIDENT MANAGEMENT—ESF INTEGRATION

The next step for the Disaster Committee is to place each ESF, along with its related agencies, into a generic incident management system. This process is not complicated. Remember the Incident Management Model:

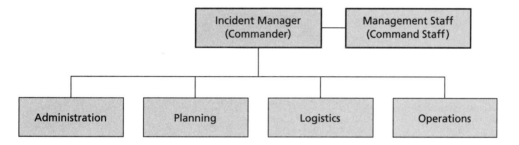

When each ESF is assigned to the appropriate section, there is an integrated system and a Disaster Plan that responds to any emergency or disaster. (See Figure 9-3.) ESF assignments can be as follows:

1. Planning
   a. ESF 5, Information and Planning
2. Logistics
   a. ESF 1, Transportation
   b. ESF 2, Communications
   c. ESF 7, Resource Support
   d. ESF 11, Food and Water
   e. ESF 12, Energy
   f. ESF 15, Volunteers and Donations
3. Operations
   a. ESF 3, Public Works
   b. ESF 4, Firefighting
   c. ESF 6, Mass Care
   d. ESF 8, Health and Medical
   e. ESF 9, Search and Rescue
   f. ESF 10, Hazardous Materials
   g. ESF 13, Military Support
   h. ESF 14, Public Information
   i. ESF 16, Law Enforcement

(NOTE: At the local level, ESF 13 coordination is via Liaison on the Management Staff.)

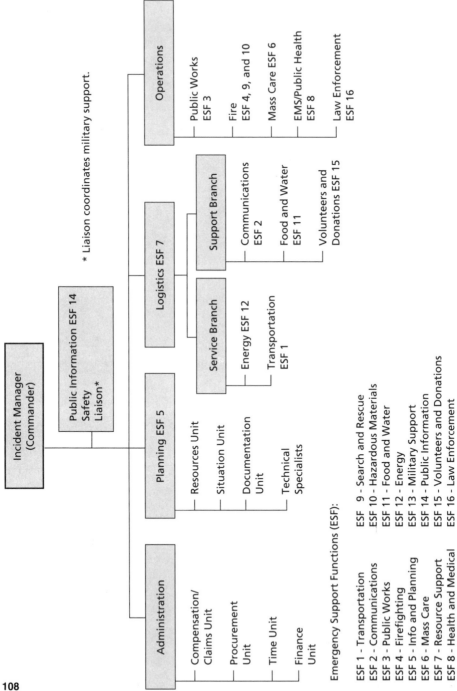

Figure 9-3
Community Disaster Planning—Interface of Federal Response Plan with Incident Management System

Emergency Support Functions (ESF):

ESF 1 - Transportation
ESF 2 - Communications
ESF 3 - Public Works
ESF 4 - Firefighting
ESF 5 - Info and Planning
ESF 6 - Mass Care
ESF 7 - Resource Support
ESF 8 - Health and Medical

ESF 9 - Search and Rescue
ESF 10 - Hazardous Materials
ESF 11 - Food and Water
ESF 12 - Energy
ESF 13 - Military Support
ESF 14 - Public Information
ESF 15 - Volunteers and Donations
ESF 16 - Law Enforcement

This alignment of ESFs and incident management functions is flexible. The Disaster Committee may decide that ESF 6 (Mass Care) is a logistics function instead of an operational one, or that military support is a planning function, and not a liaison function. The rule is, "Be flexible; if it works for the community, do it".

By aligning ESFs with the Incident Management structure, a chain of command and flow of information are provided. The relationship among ESFs is established.

Critical Factor:

The Incident Management Model is the vehicle for establishing the relationship among the ESFs.

With this system, any type of disaster is effectively managed. As problems in the disaster unfold, they are categorized as operations, logistics, planning, or administration. Because of the ESF structure, appropriate agencies, personnel, and resources are utilized as needed. NOTE: *The ESF System is not a management system/model. The ESF System identifies support agencies for the Incident Management System (IMS).*

DISASTER PLAN SUMMARY

Previous sections of this chapter presented a detailed discussion of the key steps in a Community Disaster Plan. These major points are summarized as:

1. Establish a local Disaster Committee.
2. Prepare a chart of the sixteen ESF's.
3. Determine lead agencies and support agencies for each ESF.
4. Decide where each ESF fits into the incident management structure.
5. Develop MOUs between emergency management and ESF agencies.
6. Have the Disaster Committee conduct a community threat assessment.
7. Schedule quarterly meetings of the Disaster Committee.
8. Respond to the next disaster "like you own it".

REGIONAL MEDICAL ALLIANCES

In many states, there are EMS districts organized for state administrative purposes. These regional districts usually include several counties. An EMS District is an effective group for ESF 8 planning. At district meetings, after the boring administrative issues, you can discuss disaster plans.

Specific disaster planning issues include:

- Development of common terminology.
- IMS training and implementation of the IMS.
- Establishment of disaster communications procedures, including frequencies, protocol, and transmission methods.
- Resource lists.
- Regional medical control.
- Regional medical protocol.
- Regional grant funding.

A model of an effective regional medical alliance is District I EMS in northwest Florida. The group consists of all counties in the department of health, District I. The district includes the counties of Escambia, Santa Rosa, Okaloosa, and Walton.

District I EMS meets every other month. Attendees include hospital representatives, medical directors, and EMS representatives. A district protocol and trauma transport protocol are in place. Baptist Hospital Lifeflight (Pensacola) coordinates helicopter air ambulance protocol.

The Medical Incident Management System is to be used for all disaster operations. Regional logistics support uses disaster caches. Each county has a two-case cache of BLS supplies that can treat up to fifty patients. These caches can be quickly transported to a nearby county for mutual aid.

Medical Control is assigned to the Lifeflight Dispatch Center. Lifeflight maintains a call roster of all emergency EMS agencies. It also monitors regional bed status and coordinates air ambulance operations.

The District I EMS group was tested when a U.S. Air Force C-141 cargo plane crashed in a nighttime rainstorm near Hurlburt Field in Fort Walton Beach, Florida. Twelve ALS ambulances were mobilized from a three county area and staged at the crash site. Unfortunately, all nine crew members on the aircraft died on impact.

A Disaster Medical Assistance Team (DMAT), formed by District I, responded to Miami after Hurricane Andrew. The DMAT performed exemplary service during the nine days of operations. (See Chapter 12.)

In 1994, District I EMS received a grant from the State of Florida to develop a regional response trailer. The trailer is maintained by the DMAT. It is fully stocked with medical supplies, generators, tents, and a command box. The forward portion of the trailer is an air conditioned command center. The unit has a communications repeater, handheld radios, and antennas on a roof platform. This unit can be towed by a pickup truck to any regional disaster, or be airlifted to any location.

District I EMS sponsors a yearly trauma conference. The two-day conference includes national level speakers on disaster and emergency medicine. Proceeds from the conference are used for fund matching of state grants and other viable medical projects. The annual District I Trauma Conference provides great training and excellent networking, and continues to grow.

MAJOR EVENT PLANNING

The IMS is a reactive system; a disaster occurs, somebody calls 9-1-1, and the reaction begins. The IMS can also be proactive. For major scheduled events, the tools in the IMS are used to anticipate problems and plan for them.

Many agencies have used the IMS Model to effectively plan for the Indianapolis 500, the 1996 Olympics (Atlanta), a Hell's Angels convention, national political conventions, and air shows. Sarasota County, Florida Emergency Management uses the IMS to plan for the annual offshore powerboat races.

Think about the IMS boilerplate: Management, Operations, Logistics, Planning, and Administration. Every major event will have problem areas that center around coordination (Management), Operations, and Logistics.

The first step is to identify the Incident Manager and the Management Staff. There may be several Incident Managers if a unified structure is feasible. The liaison position is essential because of the large number of cooperating and assisting agencies (separate from ESF Agencies) that are involved in an event or festival. The Public Information slot is needed to communicate with the public, give injury prevention information, and coordinate with the public relations efforts of event sponsors. A Safety Officer ensures that all plans are safe. The TIPS component is nice, but not essential. (Hopefully, things will go well and people won't need stress intervention.)

Operations is the big player in this game. An early step is to identify the operational problems and the related ESFs that will respond. Each ESF must then identify its own operational concerns. For example: ESF 8 (Medical) has to ask the following questions:

1. What are the potential medical hazards of the event?
2. How many patients can be expected?
3. How many BLS treatment areas are needed and where? How about ALS?
4. How will units and treatment areas be staffed?
5. What transportation assets (ground, air, and water) will be needed?
6. What receiving facilities will be involved?
7. What first responder agencies will be needed to support ESF 8?
8. Where will vehicles be staged?

As always, Logistics will closely follow Operations. In the plan, the operational agencies will need continuous logistical support. Identify the service and support needs, and assign ESFs and their related agencies to the service and support branch. A crucial support ESF is Communications. Address the issue of dozens of agencies, spread over a large area, having to talk to each other. Consider networks other than handheld RF, such as cellular, portable fax, and computer networks.

Logistics questions for ESF 8 are:

1. What communication networks are available? How about radio caches?
2. What are sources of BLS/ALS supplies? What about disaster caches?

3. Where is the fuel supply?
4. Will there be a need for food, water, and facilities?

The Planning Section has to work with all sections to orchestrate the overall product, an effective plan. The Planning Section must ensure that an Incident Action Plan (IAP) is communicated and written in an understandable format. The Planning Section, during the event, must monitor all incidents and restructure operational plans in real time. They must also provide weather information, track resources, maintain situation status boards, and properly document IMS functions. A major function of the documents unit will be the gathering of patient records and statistical reports for post-incident analysis.

Lastly is Administration, with the major component of this section being finance. Finance must ask the hard questions: Who is paid; who is a volunteer? Can we afford the overall plan? What services will be reimbursed, and by whom? What contracts or MOUs will be needed?

The most difficult aspect of major event planning is estimating the number of patients. Weather is always a factor in outdoor events. Extreme heat, thunderstorms, and cold are conditions that create patients. In the Pope's 1993 visit to Denver, patient estimates were exceeded tenfold because of extremely hot weather. Drugs and alcohol are a negative influence. (Rock concerts are less than drug-free.)

Plan for an MCI during an event. In the Ramstein Air Show, an acrobatic aircraft team crashed into the crowd. At an Indianapolis 500, there was a collapse of a large section of bleachers. There have been cases of propane tank explosions at events and festivals. Terrorism is a possibility, especially if national or international political leaders are part of the event. Protests such as we have witnessed at political events or abortion clinics also portend problems.

If there is a moderate to high potential for an MCI, a disaster task force should be staged for immediate response. A DMAT is an excellent source of people and expertise. The task force should have a command box, disaster caches, communications equipment, and vehicles (air or ground) for quick response.

Major event planning is now a module in the Incident Management System (IMS) National Training Curriculum. Important steps in major event planning are summarized as follows:

1. Establish an early liaison with the major sponsoring agency or organizations.
2. Pick the management team.
3. Establish a Planning Committee, with someone assigned to Operations, Logistics, Planning, and Administration.
4. Assign ESF agencies to the four major sections.
5. Write a comprehensive Incident Action Plan (IAP).
6. Develop contracts or MOUs with cooperating and assisting agencies.
7. Estimate the number of potential patients using the SWAG (simple wild-assed guess) method.
8. Make sure the plan is adequately financed.
9. Use public information effectively.

10. Plan for an MCI task force.
11. Have a post-event analysis meeting, and prepare a post-event report.

DISASTER HISTORY—WHAT WAS LEARNED

In disaster planning, a knowledge of previous disasters can prevent making the same mistakes again. Make every effort to read the literature after action reports and incident critiques of any type disaster that may threaten the area. The Internet is a source of post-incident information. Videotape is available from news sources and commercial producers of EMS videos.

Every disaster is different, yet there are common threads. A summary of major problems from disasters over the past fifty years are as follows:

1. Communications suffer from instant overload. Radio traffic is utter chaos. Key units cannot get an open channel; urgent messages are lost.
2. Vehicle traffic near the scene is gridlocked. Sightseers and emergency units block all roads.
3. Supplies are almost immediately depleted. Logistics becomes a continuous problem that lasts throughout the incident (days or weeks).
4. The right patients do not get to the right medical facility. The nearest hospital gets slammed, while other facilities receive few patients. Some patients are transported by private vehicles.
5. Freelance emergency units respond from long distances. These units often cause severe traffic and coordination problems. Initially, there is a shortage of emergency vehicles; later, vehicles are wall-to-wall.
6. Human services, especially in natural disasters, are neglected or slow to respond. Victims need shelter, food, clothing, and financial assistance.
7. There is a major fatigue factor for rescuers. The need for sleep periods and crew rotation is not recognized until people begin to "crash" from lack of sleep.
8. The media blitzes the scene; media vehicles are plentiful; telephone lines and cellular channels become overloaded. There are never enough PIO people to feed the media.
9. Dispatch centers and emergency management offices are overwhelmed with telephone calls. There are not enough lines or people to handle the call volume.
10. The emotional toll on emergency personnel is high. The mental stress is never fully appreciated until people begin to break down. TIPS personnel are often inadequate and may also become emotionally stressed.

SUMMARY

Disaster planning should begin by establishing a Disaster Committee. Response agencies, and agencies that support emergency operations, should be Disaster Committee members. The Department of Emergency Management organizes the committee.

Each community is vulnerable to many types of disasters. The Disaster Committee conducts a community disaster study to uncover vulnerable areas of concern.

The Federal Response Plan has identified Emergency Support Functions (ESFs). Many states and local governments have adopted ESFs. Each ESF has a lead agency and many support agencies. Health and Medical is ESF 8. The Disaster Committee identifies all local agencies applicable to each ESF.

The ESFs are then integrated with the Incident Management System (IMS) format. Each ESF is assigned to Operations, Logistics, Planning, and Administration. The IMS is the model that dictates coordination and information flow among ESFs, combining the ESFs with IMS results in a Community Disaster Plan that applies to any incident.

Regional medical alliances are effective groups for emergency planning and response. They develop regional medical and communications protocols, training/implementation of the IMS, resource lists, and regional medical control, and serve as a vehicle for grants. The medical alliance can further extend activities by sponsoring a DMAT and/or emergency medical conferences.

Major event planning is an important element in a Community Disaster Plan. Mass spectator events such as festivals, rock concerts, sporting events, and religious gatherings are potential mass casualty incidents. The IMS is a boilerplate for an effective scheduled event plan. The plan begins by identifying a management team and establishing liaison with the event sponsors or event coordinating agencies. Operations, Logistics, Planning, and Administration sections are identified. ESFs are identified and assigned to the appropriate section in the IMS. These actions are the basis for the Incident Action Plan (IAP). An MCI task force should address the mass casualty issue. Lastly, a post-event analysis should be conducted, and an after-action report should be written.

Be a good disaster planner by being a disaster student. Study books, articles, post-incident reports, and videos of major incidents. High-impact EMS incidents share common threads, including communications systems overload, heavy vehicle traffic, fast resource depletion, the wrong patients going to the wrong facilities, a lack of appreciation for human services needs, a need for personnel rest periods and rehabilitation, freelance response agencies, a media blitz, overloaded dispatch centers, and a high emotional toll on rescuers and care givers.

CHAPTER QUESTIONS/EXERCISES

1. Establish a Disaster Committee, or use the agency to complete the Community Threat Assessment form (Figure 9-1) in the text. What disaster potentials were uncovered that have not been planned?
2. Discuss and define the concept of Emergency Support Functions (ESF).
3. List the sixteen ESFs. Identify a lead agency and support agencies or organizations in your community or region for each ESF.
4. Discuss ESF/IMS integration. Determine where each ESF fits into the Incident Management System.

5. List and discuss the elements of an effective Disaster Plan.

6. What are the steps in developing a major event Incident Action Plan (IAP)?

7. Great news! You've just been informed that next year's Republican National Convention will be held in your city, and you'll be the Incident Manager. Identify the following problems:

   a. What is the potential for an MCI?
   b. What are the ESFs and their related agencies?
   c. What regional, state, and federal assistance will be needed?
   d. What financial costs will impact the plan?
   e. How would the number of patients be estimated?

8. List and discuss at least four major problem areas that seem to occur in most high-impact EMS incidents.

10

RESPONSE AGENCY MANAGEMENT SYSTEMS

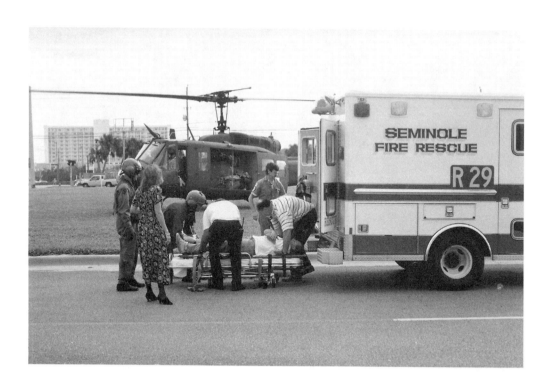

Chapter Objectives

After reading this chapter, you will be able to accomplish the following objectives:

1. Understand the integration of response agency management systems into the Medical Incident Management System.
2. Describe the relationship of an EMS unit to various incident management systems.
3. Diagram the Public Works ICS and discuss its major components.
4. Diagram the Fire ICS and discuss its major components.
5. Diagram the Law Enforcement ICS and discuss its major components.
6. Diagram the Hospital Emergency ICS and discuss its major components.
7. Understand how a medical unit can evolve into an IMS operations structure.
8. Describe the concept of EOC/ICS integration.

RESPONSE AGENCY MANAGEMENT SYSTEMS

The EMS/IMS is structured for mass casualty incidents. However, there are many emergency incidents that do not involve multiple patient injuries, but they always exist. These incidents include industrial disasters, public works operations, law enforcement incidents, and firefighting. There is also an incident management system that provides an organization for hospital disasters.

All of the Incident Management Systems (still referred to as the Incident Command System, ICS, in some agencies) have the same principles discussed in Chapter 1. These principles include unity of command, span of control, an incident action plan, common terminology, effective coordination, and logistical support. In each system, the basic structure is a Management Staff that supervises an Operations Section, Logistics Section, Planning Section, and Administration Section. These systems also have a common management structure that provides division into branches (branch director), sectors (group/division), strike teams or task forces (strike team leader), and finally units (unit leader).

EMS UNITS IN OTHER SYSTEMS

The agency-specific management systems (hospital IMS is an exception) all have an EMS unit assigned to the Logistics Section, Support Branch. The purpose of the medical unit is to treat operations personnel or civilian victims. The medical unit was first structured in the wildland fire ICS, where the EMS unit is used to evaluate, treat, and transport injured firefighters. In the structural fire ICS, EMS units are in the standby mode at fire scenes. Similar support is utilized at law enforcement, public works, or industrial incidents.

If the incident escalates to the MCI level, additional EMS units or EMS strike teams are utilized. When the incident escalates to a long-term MCI level, a major change must occur. Medical concerns no longer remain a support function in the Logistics Section. Medical care becomes an operations function. This requires the establishment of an EMS Branch in the Operations Section. The change reflects the evolving nature of the incident. Instead of the problem being purely fire, law enforcement, or public works, the EMS aspects now have equal footing.

The EMS unit leader has the burden of initiating escalation of EMS functions to an Operations Section (branch level status.) The system builds from the ground up. When the medical unit or EMS strike team leaders get overwhelmed, they must notify the Incident Manager, via their Logistics Section Chief, of the need for a change. (It's time to dig deeper into the IMS toolbox.)

The EMS unit leader is elevated to a Branch Director, or other people in the EMS chain of command are called to assume this position. The EMS Branch Director, in coordination with the Operations Section Chief and the Incident Manager, will then establish a treatment sector, a triage sector, and a transportation sector (see Figure 10-1).

EMS units do not form a separate management system. Instead, they integrate with the established IMS. Because of the common rules and common terminology in IMS, this integration is quick and effective.

The EMS function is downsized in a similar manner. Patient care may be under control, but other operational units may need to function for some time. Where there is no need for an EMS Branch, the EMS system is reduced back to an EMS unit.

The two important concepts discussed are:

1. Medical functions integrate into the IMS structure: EMS units form an EMS Incident Management System, under an EMS Branch, not a separate system.
2. EMS functions escalate from unit level to branch level, or vice versa, as the incident evolves.

An urban structural fire demonstrates the changing incident management structure. When a working fire is declared, an EMS unit responds for standby purposes. The EMS team reports to the Logistics Section. Initially, two victims are treated for smoke inhalation and transported. A secondary search uncovers four patients. More EMS units respond, with a supervisor to lead an EMS strike team. There is fire

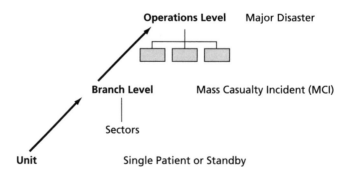

Figure 10-1 Expansion of EMS/IMS

extension into an occupied exposure, and a structural collapse. There are now six injured firefighters and ten civilian victims. The EMS strike team leader declares an MCI. The EMS Director responds and becomes the EMS Branch Director. He/she then establishes the appropriate IMS structure.

Later, the fire is controlled. All patients have been transported, and fire overhaul is underway. The IMS is demobilized with a single EMS unit remaining on the scene in a standby mode.

THE FIRE INCIDENT COMMAND SYSTEM (ICS)

The IMS model for all agencies was derived from the wildland fire ICS. The operations objective in the fire ICS is fire suppression. The Operations Section is divided into a Ground Operations Branch and Air Operations Branch.

The Ground Operations Branch consists of engines, tenders, and fire teams that are organized as single resources, task forces, or strike teams.

Air Operations are very intricate on wildland fires, and are organized as a branch level status. This branch is further divided into an air support group and an air attack group. On major fires, there is a combination of fixed wing aircraft and helicopters dropping water at precise locations. This requires water pickup locations, helibases, heliports, and fixed wing bases, all coordinated by an air traffic control system.

Since wildland fires usually occur in remote locations, the Logistics Section uses a fully staffed Service Branch and Support Branch. These branches provide a food unit and facilities unit. A medical unit is also assigned to the Service Branch.

The structural firefighting system is called the National Fire Service Incident Management System (Fire IMS). (See Figure 10-2.) It uses the same boilerplate as the wildland system, but operations branches are divided differently. The Fire Branch consists of divisions/groups of units, strike teams, and task forces. This is the most commonly used branch. The Haz Mat Branch is initiated for hazardous materials problems or chemical/biological terrorism. A Mass Casualty Branch is initiated if the incident becomes an MCI. In this case (as previously discussed), medical treatment is elevated to branch status and is commanded by an EMS Fire Chief, or a third service EMS manager, using the IMS.

Communications needs are met by using several tactical channels. The Fire Branch, EMS Branch, and Haz Mat Branch are assigned separate tactical channels. In major incidents, there may be logistics and air operations tactical channels.

In the Fire IMS, the medical unit is assigned to firefighter rehabilitation (rehab) during operations where mass casualties are not a factor. Treating firefighters is a challenge because they have a "testosterone moral code," which means you fight until you drop. Female firefighters have a similar "estrogen code." In summary, good luck when treating firefighters.

The most common interface between Fire and EMS is during motor vehicle accidents. Fire is assigned the duties of rescue/extrication and control of fuel spills

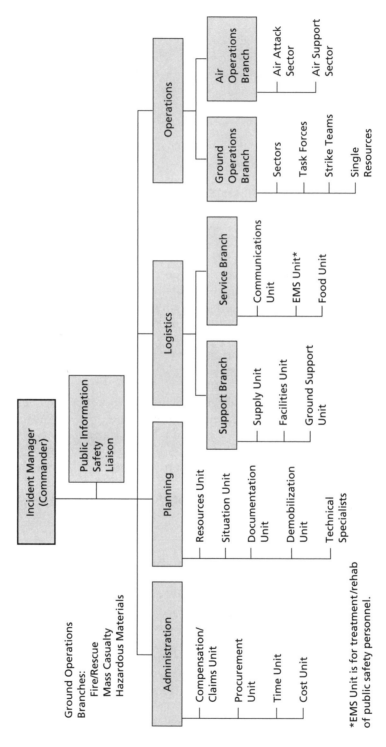

Ground Operations
Branches:
Fire/Rescue
Mass Casualty
Hazardous Materials

*EMS Unit is for treatment/rehab
of public safety personnel.

Figure 10-2 National Fire Service IMS—Major Incident

and fire. EMS is assigned the duties of patient care and transport. If the incident is an MCI, an EMS Branch Director will supervise a treatment sector, triage sector, and transportation sector.

MANAGEMENT OF INDUSTRIAL DISASTERS

In many areas of the country, there are industrial operations that rival a small city in size and complexity. This includes mines, plants, factories, refineries, and chemical companies. These organizations are vulnerable to natural disasters, explosions, fires, major haz mat spills, and terrorism.

Industry maintains private response teams called Plant Emergency Organizations (PEOs). (They were previously called Industrial Fire Brigades.) PEOs have trained emergency teams for fire suppression, confined space rescue, elevated rescue, and chemical spill suppression. The PEO coordinates with in-plant security and medical teams. (See Figure 10-3.)

In the Industrial IMS, the Operations Section is divided into the PEO, Medical, and Plant Maintenance Branches. The Plant Maintenance Branch has functions similar to a Public Works Branch in a government structure. Security is usually a support function. If the incident requires law enforcement, security moves to branch status in the Operations Section.

In industrial disasters, it is very important for the PEO and other industrial segments to effectively integrate with local government agencies. Industrial companies rarely have the resources to handle a plant disaster without mutual aid. Effective integration is assured when agencies on both sides of the fence use the IMS structure. Because of common organization and common terminology, the IMS becomes a valuable asset.

Industrial accidents present serious medical challenges to EMS units or strike teams. There may be burn cases and chemical injuries, along with multisystem trauma. Patients may be in hot zones and require rescue by the PEO or firefighters before triage and treatment. Patient decon may be necessary. (See Chapter 8.)

Technical advisors are an important asset in industrial emergencies. Patients can be injured by industrial processes or special chemicals unfamiliar to paramedics. Industrial hygienists, chemists, engineers, and safety inspectors, available from the industrial staff, can provide life-saving technical assistance.

Trauma intervention is another important asset to the EMS Branch. Industrial MCIs generate a flood of relatives and friends responding to the scene. These people are directed to an area distant from treatment and transportation areas. TIPs personnel have a calming affect on family members awaiting news about casualties.

122

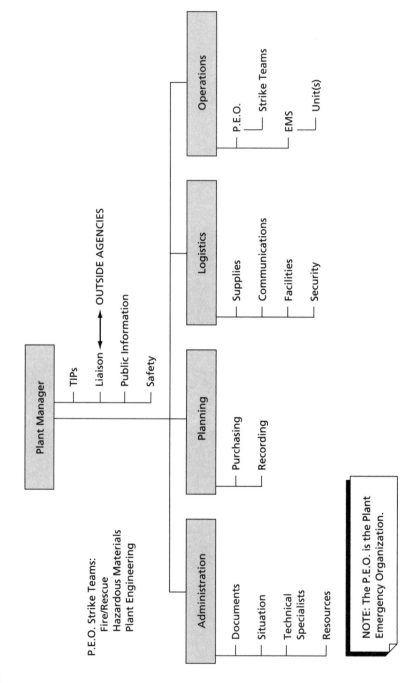

Figure 10-3 Industrial Incident Command System

LAW ENFORCEMENT INCIDENT COMMAND

The Law Enforcement Incident Command System (LEICS), like other systems, is an extension of the IMS. Progression of a LEICS has been slower than the fire service or emergency medical services command system because of the nature of law enforcement operations. Normally, police/security incidents involve one or two units. In the past, law enforcement agencies had limited experience in large-scale operations involving large numbers of personnel, vehicles, and multi-faceted mission objectives. Recent history has required law enforcement agencies to prepare for large-scale incidents.

Major incidents include natural disasters, transportation accidents, mass shooting incidents, bombings, hostage situations, and terrorism. Many of these incidents result in prolonged operations, military in nature.

LEICS divides mission assignments into groups/divisions. (See Figure 10-4.) These assignments include units and/or tactical teams. The primary groups/divisions are SERT (Special Emergency Response Team), hostage negotiation, bomb disposal, traffic control, and evacuation. The structure discussed is oriented to ground operations. Law enforcement agencies that have air assets assign an Air Operations Branch, similar to the fire organization.

The Logistics Section is divided into three groups. The service group has a communications unit, a food unit, and a medical unit. The supplies group has a ground support unit, a staging unit, and a supply unit. The personnel group has a volunteer services unit and a mutual aid unit (Figure 10-4).

The Planning Section in LEICS is called a Plan/Intel Section. Intel means intelligence and is responsible for intelligence information on hostages, suspects, terrorists, or other aspects of an incident.

EMS is at risk in law enforcement scenarios. EMS units, arriving with first response officers, may be threatened with gunfire. The EMS unit leader must determine the hot zone, and stage in a safe area, secured by a law enforcement perimeter. EMS units have to be prepared to move quickly if their staging area comes under fire. It is emotionally difficult for EMS units to remain staged when they know there are patients. But the temptation to "charge" must be resisted to ensure safety. In many areas, EMS maintains "SWAT Medic" teams that are specially trained to support law enforcement.

The trauma from law enforcement incidents can be hideous. Victims may be severely injured from explosives and military type weapons. There may also be a need to decontaminate officers exposed to chem-bio weapons.

PUBLIC WORKS INCIDENT COMMAND

After the experience with Hurricane Hugo, and scores of other natural disasters, the American Public Works Association adopted the IMS model. The end product was the Public Works IMS. (See Figure 10-5.) This system was implemented with a training program and mailed to public works agencies throughout the United States. The

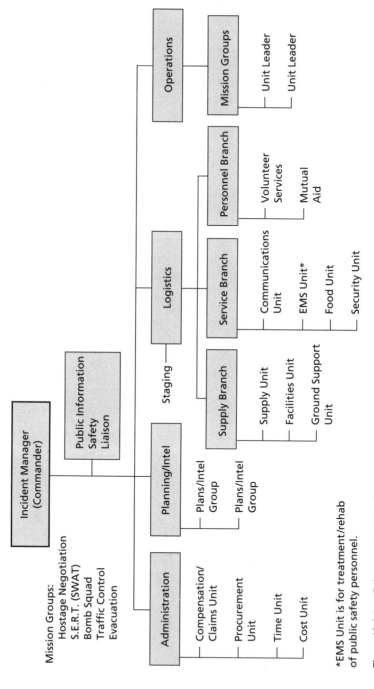

Mission Groups:
Hostage Negotiation
S.E.R.T. (SWAT)
Bomb Squad
Traffic Control
Evacuation

*EMS Unit is for treatment/rehab of public safety personnel.

Figure 10-4 Law Enforcement Incident Command System (LEICS)—Major Incident

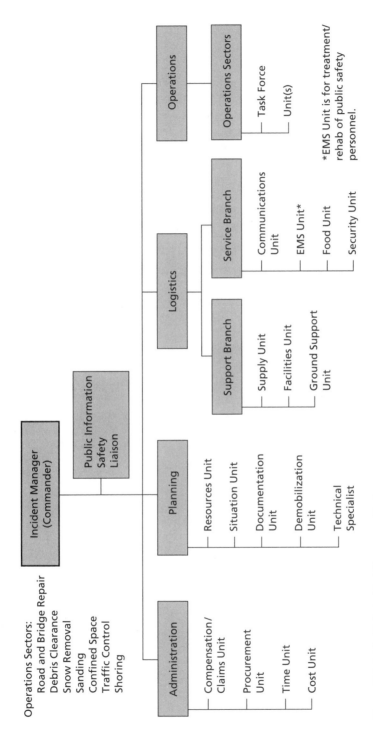

Figure 10-5 Public Works Incident Management System

125

objective of the program was to adopt a system that was operationally efficient and integrated with emergency agencies.

The primary operational objectives of public works agencies are sanding, road clearance, debris removal, diking, bridge/road repair, snow removal, confined space entry, shoring, trenching, and traffic control. These functions are carried out by personnel, units, strike teams, and task forces. For example, a debris-clearing task force might include three dump trucks, a front loader, and a team leader. All functions are assigned as groups/divisions in the Operations Section.

Public works may be a branch supporting other response agencies. This could include Haz Mat diking, clearing debris in a rescue operation, or building a road to an inaccessible site.

Routine public works operations do not require an EMS unit. During emergency operations, EMS units are usually on-scene supporting other operations.

EMERGENCY OPERATIONS CENTER INTERFACE

Major incidents require the coordination of multiple response agencies and many support agencies. In a natural disaster, all sixteen ESFs may have to function in a coordinated manner. This coordination is the responsibility of the Director of Emergency Management, and takes place at the local or county government level. Major incident operations are coordinated at an Emergency Operation Center (EOC). The EOC, also called a Multi-Agency Coordination Center (MAC), is a central command center, staffed by representatives from all sixteen ESFs (Figure 10-6).

The Operations Section consists of the following branches:

1. Medical
2. Fire/Rescue
3. Law Enforcement
4. Public Works
5. Human Services

EMS resources are coordinated at the EOC or MAC level by a senior EMS manager and the county Public Health Director. In a medical disaster, the state health department or the U.S. Public Health Service (USPHS) may respond to the region to direct all ESF 8 (Health and Medical) operations. This is accomplished by a medical support unit (MSU). The MSU is not a "unit" in incident management terminology. It is a branch level team, structured to manage ESF 8 functions. The MSU may operate in the EOC or locate in another building, if there are space limitations.

In this book, discussion has focused on emergency medical operations. In a medical disaster, functions expand to include community health issues such as:

1. Assessment of health/medical needs
2. Health surveillance
3. Medical care personnel
4. Health/medical equipment and supplies
5. Patient evacuation

6. In-hospital care
7. Food/drug medical service safety
8. Worker health/safety
9. Radiological hazards
10. Chemical hazards
11. Biological hazards
12. Mental health
13. Public health information
14. Vector control (control of disease-carrying organisms, usually rodents)
15. Potable water/waste water and solid waste disposal
16. Victim identification/mortuary services.

All of these functions are assigned as a branch, group/division, or unit in the IMS.

In a medical disaster, all ESF 8 functions are not at one location. Each geographic area where medical functions are conducted is a separate "incident," related to the "big incident." Each incident has an Incident Manager and an IMS. These Incident Managers report to the EOC or MSU. The EOC or MSU maintains the big picture and coordinates ESF functions coming from state or federal sources.

An earthquake serves as an example. The disaster is a medical disaster. Medical problems include:

1. A school collapse with trapped students.
2. A severely damaged hospital.

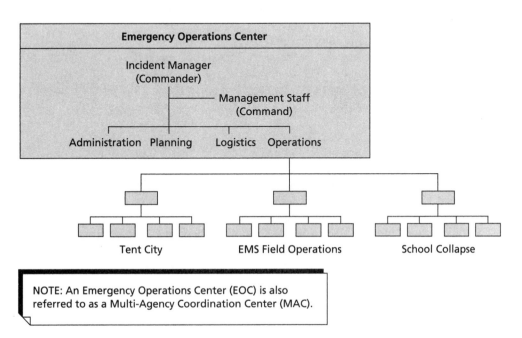

NOTE: An Emergency Operations Center (EOC) is also referred to as a Multi-Agency Coordination Center (MAC).

Figure 10-6 Emergency Operations Center Interface With Emergency Medical Services

3. A large volume of emergency calls.

4. A large tent city of homeless victims.

The school collapse has a Fire Chief Incident Manager. EMS is an Operations Branch. The hospital operates as a clinic in a nearby undamaged building staffed by a DMAT. The emergency calls are managed by the EMS Director at the EOC. The tent city is managed by a Public Health Officer.

Each "incident" in this scenario has its own IMS structure. Any medical support requests are channelled to the MSU. These requests are routed to the MSU Operations, Logistics, Planning, or Administration Section, or the Management Staff. The appropriate ESF then receives the mission request and reacts accordingly. If an ESF has inadequate resources (a likely situation), the applicable state or federal ESFs are tasked.

This process develops from a simple structure; functions are conducted at the lowest level. Additional needs channel upward from a unit all the way to an MSU controlling federal resources. *The critical factor is that the IMS structure is maintained at all levels in a medical disaster.*

HOSPITAL EMERGENCY INCIDENT COMMAND SYSTEM (HEICS)

In 1991, the Orange County Health Care Agency Emergency Medical Services received a grant from the California Emergency Medical Services Authority to develop the Hospital Emergency Incident Command System (HEICS). Orange County EMS produced a document that includes an organizational chart and job action sheets (position descriptions). (See Figure 10-7.)

The HEICS uses the national IMS structure, common terminology, and standard procedures. The HEICS is designed for any hospital emergency. This includes external emergencies such as terrorism, MCIs or medical disasters, or internal emergencies such as fires, explosions, Haz Mat, mass shootings, or natural disasters.

The organizational chart for the HEICS appears complex, but close examination reveals a familiar pattern. There is a Management Staff supervising the four major IMS sections. The Operations Section has three branches. A reminder: The functions and units in the HEICS are tools. Full use of this chart would require the staff of a large hospital; the incident would be a "once in a career" event. Each tool is used as needed, and discarded after utilization. Remember that one person can also be responsible for two or more functional assignments.

At the management level, the Liaison Officer is an important position. A scenario large enough to cause the HEICS to be implemented is a scenario requiring outside agencies. In a medical disaster, the Liaison Officer interacts with the county EOC and/or a state/federal MSU. (See Chapter 12, Hurricane Andrew.)

The Operations Branches are Medical Care, Ancillary Services, and Human Services. Medical Care is the largest branch and is divided into an inpatient services

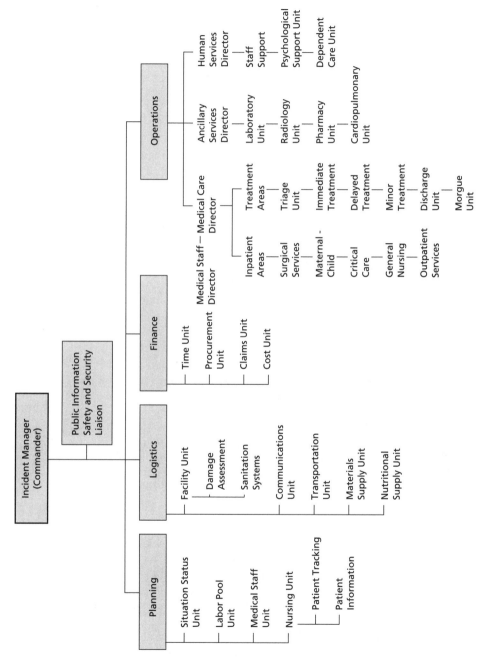

Figure 10-7 Hospital Emergency Incident Command System (HEICS)—County of Orange, Emergency Medical Services

The Operations Branches are Medical Care, Ancillary Services, and Human Services. Medical Care is the largest branch and is divided into an inpatient services group and a treatment area group. The inpatient services has units as follows:

1. Surgical services unit
2. Maternal-child unit
3. Critical care unit
4. General nursing care unit
5. Outpatient services unit

The treatment group is organized using the IMS structure as follows:

1. Triage unit
2. Immediate treatment unit
3. Delayed treatment unit
4. Minor treatment unit
5. Discharge unit
6. Morgue unit

The Ancillary Services Branch has radiology, laboratory, pharmacy, and cardiopulmonary units. The Human Services Branch has staff support, psychological support, and dependent care units.

In the HEICS, the transportation unit is assigned to the Logistics Section. The transportation unit coordinates internal transportation of patients and transport of discharged patients. In an internal disaster, the hospital is the source of victims and may have to transport patients to other hospitals.

The HEICS is an important planning and emergency response guide for medical facilities. The HEICS provides effective liaison with outside agencies that are trained in the Incident Management System. Further, the HEICS is a combination of hospital positions with the IMS that provides an efficient organization for managing a hospital disaster.

MILITARY LIAISON

In many communities, there are military bases that have emergency response agencies. These agencies are frequently used for mutual aid by the civilian community. Vice versa, civilian agencies are used as resources for on-base incidents.

In past years, coordination between military and civilian emergency response agencies was ineffective. Command structure, terminology, and procedures were incompatible. This unfortunate situation has changed. In the early 1990s, the U.S. Air Force mandated that all response agencies in the Air Force implement IMS (U.S. Air Force Ops Plan 355.1). The Air Force Fire Service was the first agency to complete the transition. Coordination problems have been reduced or eliminated because agencies on both sides of the military fence are wearing the same command vests, speaking an identical language, and using common procedures. Because of IMS, people are working together.

SUMMARY

The original fire service ICS has evolved into an Incident Management System (IMS) used by all types of response agencies. There is the Fire IMS (wildland and structural), Industrial IMS, Law Enforcement ICS (LEICS), Public Works ICS, and the Emergency Operations Center (EOC) interface.

In each system, there is a medical unit for rehab and patient treatment. As the number of patients increase, the medical function moves upward in the IMS, increasing in size to a strike team/task force, group/division, branch, and section.

In all of the systems, there is a Management Staff and an Administration, Planning, and Logistics Section. These sections, and their related units, support the operations mission.

The Hospital Emergency Incident Command System (HEICS) is a specialized IMS for hospital disasters (internal or external). Hospital services are divided into a Medical Care Branch, Ancillary Services Branch, and Human Services Branch. This system provides effective disaster planning, disaster response, and coordination with outside agencies that use an IMS structure.

The military has mandated the IMS for emergency response agencies. Civilian and military agencies, especially fire services, are now coordinating effectively because they are using similar incident management systems.

CHAPTER QUESTIONS/EXERCISES

1. List and describe at least three incident management systems other than the EMS IMS.
2. What is the function of the medical unit in the systems discussed in question 1?
3. What precautions must be taken by an EMS unit or EMS strike team in Law Enforcement Operations (LEICS)?
4. Define and discuss the functions of the EOC.
5. Define and discuss the functions of the MSU.
6. Obtain an organizational chart from a medical facility in your community or region. Design a hospital disaster response system using the HEICS model.
7. What are the functions of Health and Medical (ESF 8) in a medical catastrophe?

11

TRAINING AND IMPLEMENTATION

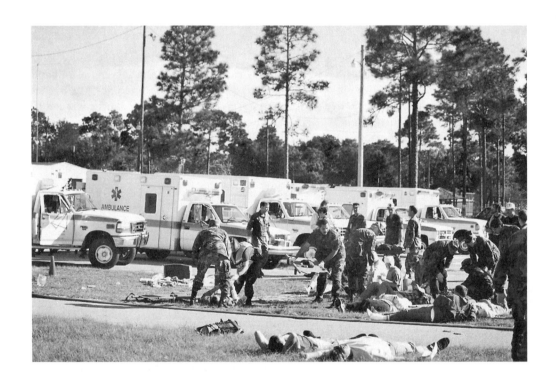

Chapter Objectives

After reading this chapter, you will be able to accomplish the following objectives:

1. Be able to design and implement an IMS training program.
2. Implement the IMS system in your agency by using the checklist at the end of this chapter.

TRAINING AND IMPLEMENTATION

The IMS is not reality until it's a routine part of your emergency medical response system. "Where do I start, and how do I do it?" are obvious questions answered in this chapter. Training and implementation are easily accomplished if you follow the procedures discussed on the following pages.

TRIAGE

Start the incident management system with triage. Triage is the IMS launching pad for several reasons. First, triage training will yield results in patient care. Second, triage will categorize patients into treatment priorities (red, yellow, green) that are the basis for the treatment sector organization of IMS. (When you triage and assign treatment categories, you have the bulk of the IMS structure.) Lastly, triage can be taught quickly to the EMS professionals and First Responders in your system.

The most effective triage program is the START system. START stands for Simple Triage And Rapid Treatment. The START system is simple, easy to learn, and applies to any MCI. This system can be taught to non-medical people in two hours. (See Figure 11-1.)

The START system is used by First Responders on all incidents with more than one patient, or used by EMS responders on an MCI. START is not intended to replace a full patient evaluation. However, at an MCI, a patient may not get a full evaluation until movement to a treatment area.

This text is not intended to be a medical care manual, but a basic discussion of START principles and its simplicity. START categorizes patients using respiration, perfusion, and mental status. The acronym is RPM.

The steps in START are:

1. Ask patients to get up and follow a responder to a safe location. Patients who respond to verbal commands and can walk are categorized as Green.
2. a. Respirations are counted. If respirations are zero, an attempt is made to establish a BLS airway by the head-tilt method. If respirations begin, the patient is Red; if no respiration, the patient is Black. (Codes are not worked in an MCI.)
   b. If respirations are greater than thirty (>30) on initial observation, patient is Red; if less than thirty(<30), patient is Yellow.
3. Perfusion is measured by capillary refill. If refill is two seconds or longer (>2), patient is Red; if less than two seconds (<2), patient is Yellow. (NOTE: Many agencies advocate the detection of a radial pulse to indicate perfusion.)

GREEN — Walks and follows commands.

RED — Respirations greater than 30;
capillary refill 2 sec. or longer;
mental confusion or no response.

YELLOW — Cannot walk; respirations
less than 30; capillary refill less than
2 sec.; responds to questions.

BLACK—Patient with no respirations
after one attempt to manually establish
an airway.

S.T.A.R.T. Card (back)

S.T.A.R.T. TRIAGE STEPS:

1. "If you can get up and walk, follow
   me."

2. Respiration
       Perfusion
           Mental status

3. "THIRTY & TWO, CAN DO."

S.T.A.R.T. Card (front)

Figure 11-1 The START Triage Card

4. Mental status is determined by asking simple questions. No response or mental confusion indicates a Red patient; a proper response is a Yellow patient.

The START training program begins by a simple explanation of the triage categories, RPM, and the START video. This requires one hour. In the second hour, each student conducts a simulated START on at least five student victims who act out each category. Before the simulation begins, demonstrate 30 respirations per minute so students can recognize rapid respiration. With thirty minutes practice, students are able to triage simulated patients in less than thirty seconds per patient. (NOTE: One student has suggested the saying, "Thirty and Two, can do!" The word thirty relates to respiration; two relates to capillary refill; "can do" to mental status.)

> **Critical Factor:**
>
> Begin IMS implementation by training all responders in the START system.

When students complete the course, they are issued a wallet-sized plastic card. On one side is a brief description of the patient categories and the criteria for respiration, perfusion, and mental status. On the reverse side are the bold letters RPM and the saying "Thirty and Two, can do!" (Figure 11-1).

After training, all EMS units are issued a set of triage ribbons, triage tags, and a triage vest. Protocol should specify that, in any incident with two or more patients, the START system is used. Responders cannot remain proficient in triage if they don't do it often. Triage on little incidents ensures success on a big incident.

Triage reports should be given on radio channels at all multi-patient incidents. These reports become familiar over the radio airwaves, and do not shock everyone on the system when large patient numbers are reported for an MCI.

TRAINING SOURCES

After the triage system is operational, basic elements of the IMS are taught to response personnel. All managers need a basic course in IMS organization and terminology. (This includes EMS and non-EMS personnel.) This session teaches chain of command, span of control, nomenclature, and position description. This initial session must be generic and not apply to any specific response agency. In past years, the only course available was the Fire ICS (wildland). Because these courses were fire specific, students in other agencies had difficulty relating to IMS principles in their agency. (Many students perceived the course as a firefighting course instead of a management course.)

These basic courses can be taught by the Emergency Management Agency (EMA). EMA is often neutral, and is better received by response and support agencies. The fire service and/or EMS training officers can also provide excellent courses if they remain agency neutral when presenting the beginning modules.

After the basic organization module, EMS professionals receive the EMS/IMS module. In these sessions, students learn about each position and how it relates to the IMS system. An excellent teaching aid is the command box. At the beginning of each class, the vests, laminated checklists, and supplies are displayed as the positions are described. Student handouts include an MCI chart, position descriptions, position checklists, and position supply lists. Each student is also issued a plastic card with the IMS chart on one side and a list of the sixteen ESFs and their local agencies on the reverse side. This card is a permanent teaching aid carried in the student's back pocket.

The IMS course is completed with a simulation module. Students see an MCI video. After review, videos of actual incidents are shown. Students are asked to select the IMS positions that were used on the incident and to critique procedures witnessed on the video. This session concludes with one or more simulations. Students don vests and use checklists and a tactical radio channel for an MCI simulation. During these simulations, management principles and organization are the goals, not medical protocols. These sessions can be held in a classroom or small outside area without using vehicles or response equipment.

Upon completion, each student is issued an IMS pocket guide. The guide contains an organization chart, position descriptions, and position checklists. It also contains a section on ESF agencies and IMS definitions. This guide is kept in each unit and serves as a quick reference or study guide.

THE RED CARD SYSTEM

In the wildland fire ICS, each position in the system is taught via a nationally certified course. A student is issued a red identification card, indicating proficiency in a given area. This is known as "red carding." For example, a person may be "red carded" in logistics, communications, or safety. This card is recognized anywhere in the United States.

In the IMS, non-treatment positions should be certified by a similar system. Presently in the IMS, there is not a national system for medical "red carding", but many local, regional, and state systems have specific standards. These standards apply to positions such as EMS Branch Director, EMS supply, transportation, triage, etc. Medical positions in treatment areas are approved through state medical certification or license, and are not "red carded."

LOGISTICS

Intense logistics training is meaningless if there are no available supplies. An effective "push" supply system is the key to implementing an effective logistics system. (See Chapter 6.) Disaster caches and public disaster kits, strategically located, make any Logistics Section Chief or EMS supply unit look good.

People from your purchasing or supply delivery system are good sources for efficient logistics and/or EMS supply personnel. These people are familiar with medical supply terms and equipment. They need training in the following areas:

1. Location of caches and disaster kits; disaster supply protocols.
2. Familiarization with Emergency Management logistics sources and ESF agencies.
3. A basic knowledge of IMS procedures and communications protocol.

The military and the U.S. Forest Service are the best sources of training in logistics operations. The military has excellent books, videos, and operating procedures on field supply operations. If you are near a military base or National Guard unit, their "loggies" (logistics types) may be a great help. The National Interagency Fire Center (Boise) also sponsors courses and has an extensive library of videos and reference sources.

EXERCISE-EXERCISE-EXERCISE

With the high degree of motor vehicle accidents in most locales, MCIs are common; a medical disaster may be once in a career. You can't be good at an MCI unless you practice. Mass casualty exercises help retain proficiency in between real incidents.

Emergency management agencies should be facilitators in a medical exercise program. The Emergency Manager is trained in exercise planning, and can serve as the vehicle for coordinating multiple agencies. Many states require county emergency management agencies to have at least yearly exercises. Military support agencies have similar requirements.

An exercise begins with an exercise plan. The exercise plan is a series of objectives that each agency wants to test. Law enforcement may want to test perimeter security; fire/rescue may want to test mutual aid procedures. EMS objectives are triage, transportation, communications, or logistics.

A common mistake in an exercise plan is to test too many objectives. Pick an important objective and a secondary objective, and concentrate on a scenario that will test the two objectives.

An effective exercise, for example, may require MCI level triage and transportation of disaster caches. An attempt to test transportation and communications in the same exercise would be ambitious and present too many issues.

The exercise should be managed by an exercise controller (EC). The EC is responsible for carrying out the exercise plan and effectively conducting the exercise. The exercise controller also has exercise evaluators. The evaluators monitor the exercise players and take notes for a post-exercise critique. A Safety Officer should be present at all exercises and have the authority to correct safety violations while the exercise is in progress.

The purpose of mass casualty exercises is not to test medical treatment. Simulating ALS care and moulage of patients does not test EMS skills or build patient care proficiency. Concentrate on testing management skills, communications, patient flow, unit coordination, inter-agency coordination, mutual aid, planning, or logistics. Logistics requirements are tested by having exercise participants write supply needs for each patient on a card. The simulated supplies are tallied for future reference.

Real accidents occur during an exercise. Actual emergencies also occur. As a safety procedure, the code, "real world" is transmitted when an accident happens during exercises. This makes all players aware that a real world problem exists, and that the problem is not a simulation. In an extreme situation, an exercise may be terminated because of real world problems.

Proper follow-up is important after an exercise. A post critique meeting should be conducted within two days. The moderator of this meeting (usually the exercise controller) has a difficult job. He/she must emphasize the positive aspects of the exercise, yet allow deficiencies to be discussed. Negative aspects of performance should always be discussed tactfully. (Don't "sugar coat" deficiencies. Just be careful about how they're presented.)

Critical Factor:

Begin and end an exercise critique on a positive note. Discuss negative observations tactfully.

The final step in a successful exercise is an after-action report. This report should balance the positive and negative findings of the evaluations and the post critique meeting. This document is important because it outlines specific deficiencies and needed improvements for participating agencies.

POST INCIDENT ANALYSIS

An evaluation of an actual incident was previously called a Post Incident Critique. Many people forgot that a critique is supposed to be positive and negative; they centered on the negative. In recent years, an incident critique became known as a Post Incident Analysis.

All major incidents should be reviewed, and an after-action report should be written. The report should emphasize strengths, weaknesses, and "lessons learned."

The IMS structure is the perfect model for evaluating performance after an MCI. Each section or unit in the IMS is analyzed using the positive/negative/lesson-learned format. The first step is to draw the EMS management system as it was utilized during the incident. (Names are not important in the diagram; functions/positions are.) Each function, from the EMS Branch Director to a ground transportation unit, is analyzed. Support functions, such as EMS supply or communications, are evaluated. Relationships between agencies and IMS sectors are very important. If appropriate, ESF agencies should be evaluated. Coordination between operations sectors and the management staff are relevant.

The Post Incident Analysis provides a method for analyzing performance. The findings, especially the lessons learned, are the basis for training, new procedures, budget or personnel needs, and inter-agency coordination.

SUMMARY OF IMS IMPLEMENTATION

The EMS Incident Management System is implemented on a step-by-step basis. The investment of time and effort will pay dividends when the next MCI happens. This final section is a checklist. Each segment of this list is an implementation objective.

1. Develop a command box with position vests, laminated checklists, an IMS chart, scene tape, and writing supplies.
2. Use the command box as a teaching aid.
3. Design wall charts of your MCI organization. Post the charts in classrooms, stations, and meeting rooms.
4. Teach the START triage system to First Responders and medical personnel.
5. Issue triage vests, triage tags, and triage ribbons to all first response units.
6. Use the START system on all MCIs.
7. Develop a written protocol that specifies what agency will provide incident management on each type of incident.
8. Develop a local/regional EMS transport protocol (air and ground).
9. Identify medical control and checklists of local/regional medical facilities.
10. Develop a logistics "push" system with disaster caches and public disaster kits.
11. Identify and train EMS supply personnel.
12. Develop a communications protocol based on plain language and feedback.
13. Develop secondary and tertiary communications loops; develop a method of data transmission.
14. Establish EMS COM procedures.
15. Work with Emergency Management on establishing a Disaster Committee.
16. Use the ESF system to identify support agencies.
17. Develop a Safety Officer program.
18. Integrate with other agency management systems (Fire IMS, LEICS, HEICS, Industrial ICS, and Public Works ICS).
19. Use the IMS, in coordination with a regional medical alliance, to develop and implement a regional Disaster Plan.
20. Develop an ongoing IMS training program.
21. Use the IMS system for scheduled event planning.
22. Use the ICS forms available via the Boise NIFC or local forestry agencies. These forms (especially the Incident Action Plan form and the Resource Tracking forms) should be used for routine administrative functions as well as emergency incidents.
23. Exercise-Exercise-Exercise.
24. Conduct a Post Incident Analysis and write an after-action report after major medical incidents.

12

EMS INCIDENT MANAGEMENT IN THE REAL WORLD

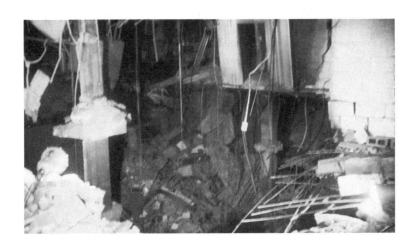

It's time to kick back after eleven chapters of academic material. This chapter is a "war story." It describes how well the IMS worked under fire, in Miami during emergency operations after Hurricane Andrew and at America's largest MCI, the New York World Trade Center bombing.

This chapter is a summary. It demonstrates how academic concepts work in the real world.

Medical Operations During Hurricane Andrew

Prepared by Hank Christen, Team Leader, Gulf Coast DMAT

Introduction

On August 29, 1992, the Gulf Coast Disaster Medical Assistance Team (DMAT) boarded the C-130 at Hurlburt Field, Florida. We were a motivated group of paramedics, nurses, doctors, firefighters, and amateur radio operators from northwest Florida. Hurricane Andrew hit Miami; it was the real thing.

The Management System

The IMS had been implemented by trial and error two years before Andrew. The basic fire ICS model was used and modified for medical operations. The teams had plenty of practice at two weekend training exercises at Keesler Air Force Base, a staged airplane crash at Pensacola Airport, and a simulated earthquake exercise at Walnut Ridge, Arkansas.

Exercises proved the management system had to be implemented as a first step. Before takeoff, critical command positions were assigned. This included issuing command vests, checklists, and handheld radios.

Experience proved to be a good teacher. We landed at Opa Locka (north Miami), approximately thirty miles north of the disaster site in Cutler Ridge (south Miami). The ground movement, with thirty-two people and all their equipment, taxed the team management system before the first patient was even treated.

The Logistics Section, commanded by Firefighter Charlie Barber, was the driving force at this point. A Mobilization Unit, formed by Firefighter Rick Moak, directed the movement of personnel and supplies. Upon arrival at Cutler Ridge, a grassy section in front of Government Center was assigned as a team home.

The mobilization unit became a facilities unit and directed the erection of tents and storing of equipment. (Capt. Richard Pitts was a great help as an electrician.) Doctors and nurses worked beside paramedics and firefighters, driving tent stakes and making beds.

We got our first lesson in flexibility upon landing. Our equipment was secured to large aluminum pallets. (They're called a 463.) The pallets are designed for Air Force transports, but are two inches too wide for Army Chinook Helicopters. We had to unload the pallets and hand load the helicopters, instead of an easy fork-lift load. When I asked an Army Sergeant about this, he replied, "That's what you get for usin' the Air Force."

Communications

We landed with radios issued to vital management units. Since MED 8 was a national mutual aid channel, radios for inter-team tactical use were set on MED 8. It was discovered that Metro-Dade Fire Rescue was using MED 8 as a dispatch channel. The communications unit carried a laptop computer with software for programming the radios. New channels were established and used throughout the incident for tactical communications.

Regional communications were another problem. The medical support unit (MSU) directed the DMATS from Government Center. When teams deployed to remote locations, problems developed. Telephones were out, and the cellular system was intermittent at best. The local public safety network was destroyed. (Metro-Dade Fire Rescue used an extended aerial ladder with a makeshift antenna attached to the tip.)

The regional problem was solved by using radio caches from the U.S. Forest Service. These VHF radios, with portable repeaters, were issued to each team and worked well.

Contacting home and the NDMS headquarters in Rockwell, Maryland, was easy. Ham operators R.W. Stancliff and Dale Sewell established a national network. This system used voice and computer packet transmissions. These channels were used for contacting families with welfare messages and for issuing press releases to Pensacola and Fort Walton Beach media.

The Incident Management System

The team received all mission assignments from the medical support unit (MSU). The MSU was headed by the overall USPHS medical commander. The MSU's job was to coordinate all ESF 8 activities. This included receiving all medical assistance requests, conducting patient needs assessment, determining medical missions, and assigning DMATs. The MSU was also responsible for logistical support of DMATs in the field.

The MSU staff was organized with an IMS structure similar to the field DMATs. There were personnel assigned to Operations, Logistics, Planning, and Administration. Military liaison was also an important MSU function. (NOTE: In IMS nomenclature, the management team is called an overhead team. The USPHS calls the overhead team an MSU.)

The mission assigned to the Gulf Coast DMAT was to relieve the Fort Wayne DMAT. Fort Wayne team leader Lynn Patton, RN, was operating an emergency room (ER) at Government Center. Two hospitals in the area were closed because of severe damage. The ER served an area of two hundred and fifty thousand people.

The change of command was not simple. It was important to interface with counterparts at every level, yet not affect patient care. This was complicated by the Fort Wayne team being physically and emotionally exhausted. Lynn and I decided to phase in the new team over a twenty-four hour period. We were assisted by EMS Director Bruce Yelverton, Assistant Team Leader.

Hurricane Andrew was the largest DMAT deployment in history. (Similar deployments would later occur for Hurricane Inniki, the Northridge Earthquake, and Hurricane Marilyn.) Other teams operating on our arrival (along with Ft. Wayne) were Albuquerque, New Mexico; Fort Thomas, Kentucky; Boston/Worcester, Massachusetts (Dr. Susan Briggs); and Winston Salem, North Carolina (Dr. Lew Stringer). Later teams that deployed into Miami were our sister team from Port Charlotte, Florida (lead by Capt. Gary Lindbergh and Connie Bowles, RN) and Toledo, Ohio, under Dr. Paul Rega, Kelly Burkholder-Allen, MPH, and Churton Budd, RN. A final DMAT deployment included DMAT stress teams from Baltimore, Maryland, and Kahului, Maui, Hawaii, along with the Tulsa, Oklahoma DMAT (Dr. Art Malone, Tim Walton.) We would later work with the Tulsa team in the Virgin Islands.

Because of the IMS, coordinating with personnel at Metro-Dade Fire Rescue was easy. When the DMAT donned identification vests for the various positions, Metro-Dade Chief Carlos Perez and his people, familiar with IMS, knew how to coordinate. Because of common terminology, people could understand communications and functions. The IMS worked just like the old wildland fire ICS. Within minutes, people from diverse agencies who had never met were efficiently doing business.

Patients were routed to a triage desk operated by Lynn McDaniels. A simple patient form included name, address, telephone number, age, sex, and a brief description of the medical complaint. The patient's triage level was indicated by a red, yellow, or green slash mark across the form with a magic marker.

There was a red, yellow, and green treatment section, with a treatment unit leader for each section. Drs. Craig Broome and Charles Neal directed the red area, nurses Patty Heath and Kay Brooks ran the yellow area, and a paramedic supervised the green section. Patients who required hospitalization were routed to a transportation unit for air or ground transport. (More about transportation later.)

We were assigned twenty-four-hour operations for nine days. I divided the team into a blue team and a gold team; each team worked a twelve-hour shift. Fatigue was a major problem. The sleep and rest area was next to the treatment area. Because of helicopter noise and emotional stress, sleep was almost impossible.

The regional medical community provided much needed support. Physicians and nurses from unaffected counties provided invaluable assistance. Pediatricians and pharmacists were especially welcomed.

The large number of medical volunteers resulted in a need for credentialing and license verification. A volunteer unit (ESF 15) was established to serve as a check-in station before volunteers were assigned to the treatment unit. Licenses were verified before patient assignments. In one case, two medical students worked for two days before it was discovered they were not physicians. (They wore scrubs and spoke the lingo.) A volunteer unit stopped the problem.

Media coverage was unrelenting. Because of personnel shortages, I doubled as the PIO. The media was escorted through treatment areas and given free access, providing patient care was not compromised. To the media's credit, this access was not abused. The coverage made the team look good to the folks back home. The highlight of the media barrage was a national feed on NBC's Today Show. I was quoted as saying,

> One afternoon, a clean cut guy in a suit entered the treatment area and identified himself as a Secret Service Agent (he fit the mold). He told me Marilyn Quayle, wife of the Vice President, would be arriving in thirty minutes. She arrived on cue, without an entourage. She was at ease with the surroundings and got the grand tour. This had a calming effect on our patients, and boosted team morale. She was a gracious lady.

Logistics

Logistics was a major lesson. Team members did not appreciate the number of logistics people required to support treatment personnel. Since people were scarce, off-duty medical personnel were used to support the working staff. The Logistics Section Chief was a busy man.

The team was advised to arrive with enough supplies and equipment to be self-sufficient for three days. This was good advice, especially for the first arriving teams.

A need for an efficient "push" logistics system was one of the major points at the post-Andrew debriefing session. In the future, a standardized cache of medical supplies, medications, and equipment will be "pushed" to the scene from regional supply depots.

DMATs ran out of cardiac monitors, monitoring pads, tetanus, insulin, suture sets, Dilantin I.V., and batteries. Local pharmacists were an enormous help. Medications were supplied by private donors and regional Veterans' Administration hospitals. There was also a need for portable refrigerators to keep insulin cold. This problem was solved by procurement from local vendors.

In remote medical areas, we were supplied by Chinook helicopters carrying sling loads. The loads included tents, blankets, cots, and non-perishable medical supplies.

Facilities were installed and maintained by the DMATs (another drain on logistics personnel). Our DMAT raised three tents in a windy rainstorm, and had an ALS treatment center operating within forty-five minutes.

Enterprising team members used plywood to construct a makeshift shower. A length of firehose, a nozzle, a hydrant wrench, and duct tape completed the project. The original shower had no roof, but a roof was built after helicopters kept flying low to watch the nurses take showers.

Water supply was another problem. The team deployed with only one day of drinking water. Fortunately, water was flowing at Government Center. The non-potable water was suitable for patient washing and irrigation. Stainless steel milk tankers supplied drinking water. In outlying areas, teams were supplied by military water buffalos (water tanks on trailers).

Patient Care

In the first three days, trauma care from storm-related injuries was the norm. Later, primary care, preventive medicine, and treatment for chronic conditions became the norm.

The most common trauma was from falls and foot injuries, as people attempted to fix their homes. Podiatrists were a big help in the suture areas. MVAs were also a constant source of trauma. Traffic was heavy, and stop lights were not functioning. There were many severe accidents caused by drivers hitting the express-way toll booths. The booths were closed, and people were not used to driving through them at high speed.

The burn cases were usually critical. Most of the burn patients were injured attempting to fill portable generators while they were running. These burns were second- and third-degree, below the waist. Most of these incidents also caused working structural fires.

Gunshot and knife trauma was down, but it didn't stop. In one case, a patient had been shot in the buttocks with a nine-millimeter pistol. He was exiting a home with a television in his hands when he was shot by the homeowner. One teenage gang member we treated had scars from eight previous gunshot wounds.

After three to four days, chronic medical problems began to surface. They included seizures, pediatric asthma, brittle diabetes, hypertension, and respiratory problems (COPD).

When large numbers of oxygen-dependent patients began to seek treatment, the yellow treatment unit was modified to include an oxygen therapy area. Large oxygen cylinders (H Cylinders) were laid on the floor, with a single hose to a manifold. The manifold supplied up to six nasal cannulas or rebreather masks. Cardboard boxes were cut on an angle and duct taped to cots to provide a means of elevating COPD patients.

Humans were not the only patients. Many homeless animals, especially dogs, wandered through the devastated areas. The dogs had lacerations from fighting, or suffered from dehydration. In a severe dehydration case, Dr. Lew Stringer started an I.V. of normal saline on a dog. Obviously, animal treatment did not compromise patient care or deplete patient supplies. Treatment of animals was well-received by the public and extended our philosophy of preservation of all forms of life.

I often think about some of the people I met during this MCI:

Eddie Miranda   He owned an oxygen therapy company in Miami. He delivered some badly needed oxygen cylinders to our team and stayed for five days.

Eddie was bilingual, and provided Spanish translation for our patients. He helped run an oxygen therapy area, second to none. When we left we gave Eddie a team tee shirt, and made him our honorary member. He was speechless, but with tears in his eyes managed to say, "I'll never forget any of you; thank you very much."

Matilda Brown   I saw her from across the room. She was a patient in the oxygen therapy unit. She wore a Panama hat, her best Sunday dress, and white shoes. "Come over here and talk to me and hold my hand, young man," she said. For a minute, I quit playing Incident Manager. We talked. She said, "Whenever I'm down, I put on my best clothes, hold my head high, and deal with life." I've thought of her many times since then.

Outreach Medicine

In a normal situation, the patient initiates access to the emergency medical system, usually via 9-1-1. In Miami, communications were malfunctioning or non-existent. It was difficult to find out who needed help, and where.

After the storm dissipated, Metro-Dade Fire Rescue had two hundred and fifty critical 9-1-1 calls holding. Fire stations in the storm area had hundreds of people reporting for medical treatment or assistance.

Each emergency run generated three more incidents. Victims were flagging down emergency vehicles responding through their neighborhood. Police units were encountering similar problems. Transit buses were also picking up patients and transporting them to treatment areas.

The public's ingenious method of accessing the medical system was breaking curfew. The dusk-to-dawn curfew was rigidly enforced by the 82nd Airborne Division and law enforcement. Any person stepping outside immediately encountered patrol units that could get medical help.

There were many freelance aid stations and treatment areas established by private medical practitioners. These units operated out of cars, tents, and motor homes. One treatment station, unknown to officials, was operated by two LPNs and a veterinarian.

When the 82nd Airborne arrived, they set up BLS aid stations at schools and parks. These areas were marked by large red balloons that were on a one-hundred-foot tether.

We were concerned that elderly patients with chronic conditions were not being treated. A similar concern existed for migrant workers in Homestead, Florida. 82nd Airborne vehicles, with DMAT members, began a house-to-house search. Many patients were found. Some were treated on site and given food, water, and essential supplies. Others were transported to a hospital, when required.

The Army used Humvees with powerful public address systems, that slowly cruised the streets and notified citizens about the location of treatment areas, supply and food areas, and information on preventive measures. The messages were broadcasted in English, Spanish, and Creole (the Haitian language).

Home health nurses played a major role. In many cases, the nurses had lost their homes and their offices. With sparse records, they attempted patient contact with personal vehicles. Many patients had left damaged homes and had to be tracked.

Patient assessment teams were sent by the MSU to survey areas and determine what care was needed. Public shelters were also assessed. As needs were uncovered, DMATs or 82nd Airborne Units were given mission assignments. The objective was to distribute medical resources in zones where they were most needed. Preventive health measures were also addressed.

Transportation

The Transportation Unit in the DMAT structure was always busy. Since emergency treatment areas could not admit patients, serious cases had to be transported to hospitals in greater Miami. Jackson Memorial Hospital (JMH), in northwest Miami, was the only operating trauma center.

A Metro-Dade firefighter was assigned to each DMAT transportation unit. When transport was required, the requests were coordinated by radio, via the firefighter.

Ground ambulances were the main transportation mode. These vehicles were Metro-Dade units, private ambulances, and ambulances from mutual aid fire departments from south and central Florida. Severe trauma cases were air evacuated to JMH. Metro-Dade's two air medical helicopters were destroyed. The flight paramedics were re-assigned to Army Black Hawk helicopters. These combined teams performed admirably. Whenever a transportation unit called for air evac, a helicopter was there within five minutes.

Response

Responding to incidents in a distant city is a strange experience. In Miami, street signs were down along with expressway exit signs. Landmarks were destroyed, making it difficult for even local units to find their way around. I am a Miami native, but still got lost.

Medical assessment teams needed maps to find their assigned areas. Helicopters had difficulty finding landing zones. In one case, helicopters couldn't find the Homestead High School football field. The field was debris littered, and did not look like a football field from the air.

Local road maps were at a premium. Government agencies quickly ran out of maps, as mutual aid and regional/national support agencies consumed the supply. The 82nd Airborne went to convenience stores to buy all the maps available. A logistics function planned for future disasters is appropriation of maps. Emergency management agencies should have at least one hundred excess maps as part of a Disaster Plan.

High technology helped solve response problems. Geo Positioning Satellite (GPS) technology was a solution. Most aircraft now have GPS navigation systems. A medical team, with an inexpensive ($500), handheld GPS receiver, can obtain exact grid coordinates and direct incoming aircraft. This is especially important at night. GPS can also be used for ground units. The course and distance to a set of coordinates can be obtained by handheld units. We did not have GPS in Miami, but GPS receivers are now required equipment. (GPS has many practical applications in day-to-day operations, especially when coordinating with helicopter air ambulances.)

Following is a vivid example of the scarcity of maps: A huge Army Chinook helicopter landed at Cutler Ridge Mall with our re-supply order. The pilot had landed at two other malls, and asked startled shoppers for directions to our site. He was relieved to finally find us. A young lieutenant remarked, "We can give you grid coordinates for the darkest back alley in Thailand, but we don't have any maps for Miami."

Geobased Information Systems (GIS) produces computer-drawn maps. The Metro-Dade County GIS Department used this effective tool to produce real-time maps of the damaged area. These maps included locations of DMATs, aid stations, water supplies, food distribution, and FEMA Disaster Assistance Centers. New maps were produced daily, giving an accurate depiction of the "big picture."

Stress Management

The trauma intervention program (TIPs) was an ongoing process. The patient care activity was like another day at the office, the environment was not. There was destruction everywhere, with no greenery. At night, the darkness was total. There were no night sounds, no crickets. Helicopter noise and sirens were all that could be heard. This environment, coupled with little or no sleep, took its toll on our patients.

The patients were in a daze, emotionally numb. The "thousand-yard stare" was common in treatment areas. People lost their homes and were suffering from injuries. Although the TIPs unit was originally slated to treat team members, their efforts were soon concentrated on patients.

Patients with injured children were devastated. In many cases, they went from numbness to hysteria without warning. The behavior affected the children and other patients. Mental health professionals became a vital facet of patient care.

Local public safety personnel reacted stoically after suffering personal losses. Firefighters, paramedics, and police officers lost their homes, yet worked long hours in the line of duty. Professionals from throughout the country conducted stress debriefings for hundreds of public safety professionals.

Our team conducted an informal debriefing after each twelve-hour shift. Team members shared feelings, talked about patients, complained about the supply bureaucracy, and bolstered each other. At the end of the session, we held hands in a moment of silence. Our intervention unit included Larry Rappe, Pat Ross, Terry Watkins, and Bill and Sandy Hartley.

Going back to the real world, post de-mobilization required an adjustment period. An arrival session was conducted at the home airport. Several weeks later we had a homecoming party where we shared pictures, jokes, and war stories. There was a comraderie that comes from dependence on others under the strain of combat.

Experience from Hurricane Andrew revealed that the mental health needs of an affected community are as serious as the trauma care needs. Mental health DMATs now exist to provide the high level of emotional care needed in a disaster area. The TIPS unit continues to be an important element in the team level management structure.

We knew that someday we might have to apply our Andrew experience at home in Florida's Panhandle. Unfortunately, 1995 was the year we were hit by Hurricane Erin. Soon after, we deployed to St. Thomas, Virgin Islands, and operated a tent emergency room for ten days. Forty-eight hours after coming home, we were hit by Hurricane Opal. We called it "Sixty Days in 95."

Summary

The IMS got a severe test in Miami, and it passed with flying colors. Patient care was effective; triage, treatment, and transport were accomplished. Interagency coordination was effective. Communications and logistics operations were strained to capacity, but remained adequate.

We had to dig deep into the IMS toolbox. For every problem, there was a solution. Most importantly, a great team of dedicated men and women, with excellent U.S.P.H.S. and VA support, performed above and beyond the call of duty.

Medical Operations at The World Trade Center Bombing © March, 1993

Prepared by D/C Paul M. Maniscalco, B.S., EMT/P, Chief of Special Operations, NYC EMS

Introduction

Terrorist acts occur worldwide, almost daily. Whether the origins are Narco-Terrorism or religious/political, we have become all too familiar with these events and the results that are perpetrated by cowardly individuals and/or organizations. As the result of a terrorist bomb on Friday, February 26, 1993, at approximately 12:18 hours, the New York City Emergency Medical Service was called upon to respond to the largest patient-generating incident in its history. No one ever imagined the scope of this incident when we commenced our response, and many people, EMS members and patients, soon had their lives changed forever.

Response

While conducting normal administrative duties at the quarters of the Special Operations Division (SOD) with Capt. Jeffrey Armstrong, S.O.D. Executive Officer, our meeting was interrupted by Lt. Robert Browne, who advised us that there was a report of a transformer explosion at the World Trade Center in lower Manhattan. We also learned that there were at least three additional calls into the 9-1-1 system corroborating the first report of an explosion.

Based on the available information, I commenced my response with Capt. Armstrong, Lt. Browne, Lt. Fenton, and the S.O.D. Emergency Response Squad (ERS). It should be noted that our (SOD) response at this juncture was predicated on the initial report of a transformer explosion. We thought the potential for a haz/mat decon was high due to the use of PCBs as transformer coolant in some locations. The Special Operations Division of NYC*EMS is responsible for patient and rescuer Haz Mat decon.

As we neared the Brooklyn Battery Tunnel, the scope of the incident started its upward growth. At this point, Lt. Juan Torres gave his preliminary report of many patients and requested numerous resources to respond. Early unconfirmed reports of a bomb began to surface. The Brooklyn Battery Tunnel was closed to all traffic except emergency vehicles, which greatly assisted the multiple responding emergency units attempting to get into lower Manhattan from the outer boroughs.

The Incident Site

To fully grasp the scope of this incident, let me digress for a moment and describe the structures and surrounding campus of the WTC complex. The World Trade Center consists of two 110-story office towers (One and Two World Trade Center), a 47-story office building (Seven World Trade Center), two nine-story office buildings (Four and Five World Trade Center), an eight-story U.S. Customhouse (Six World Trade Center), and a 22-story hotel (Vista International New York, Three World Trade Center), all of which were constructed around a five-acre plaza. All seven buildings have entrances onto the plaza, as well as on to the surrounding city streets. The Trade Center's Concourse, located immediately below the plaza, houses the largest enclosed shopping mall in Manhattan. The two office towers, each rising 1,350 feet, are the tallest buildings in New York City and the second tallest buildings in the world. The center is located on a 16-acre site in lower Manhattan, stretching from Church Street on the east to West Street on the west, and from Liberty Street on the south to Barclay and Vesey Streets on the north. The campus also has a six-level, below-grade area that accommodates over 2,000 cars for parking and provides a station and track area for the PATH (Port Authority Trans Hudson) train system. If you were to plot out the entire property horizontally, it would encompass greater than 2,000 acres. The Port Authority of New York and New Jersey reports that "some 60,000 people work in the World Trade Center, with another 90,000 business and leisure visitors coming to the center daily." The property size and numbers of people associated with the WTC Complex have qualified it for its own zip code from the U.S. Postal Service.

The Explosion, Damage, and Terrorist Group

Upon examination of the wreckage left by this bomb, FBI Special Agent David R. Williams, of the FBI Headquarters Explosives Unit, was quoted at the first press conference as saying, "This explosive device that we've seen here today is the largest by weight and by damage of any improvised explosive device since the inception of forensic explosive identification, and that's since 1925." The blast occurred on the B-2 level of the sub-basement in the underground parking structure of Three World Trade Center. The blast tore a 130-ft. × 120-ft. hole, involving 16 bays, surrounded by 20 bays of damaged eleven-inch thick, reinforced concrete slab that is "sloping up to four feet in a very precipitous state," said Leslie E. Robertson. Ms. Robertson, a World Trade Center designer, believes that the bomber was not aiming just for a parking garage and five or six people, but to take down an entire building and 25,000 workers. "It [the van] was parked right next to the outside wall of the north tower," she continued. "If you wanted to take down the towers, that would be one of the places you would try to bomb." The blast pattern extended vertically two floors through the B-1 level upward into a restaurant area of the Vista International Hotel and downward three stories to the B-5 level. The blast concussion vented itself horizontally with a massive displacement of air through the parking garage and ramps located throughout the sub-grade structure. A significant level of damage is associated with this air displacement. Numerous vehicles were picked up and tossed as they were caught in the violent air drafts. Debris flew through the air literally sandblasting items down to their bare metal. Additional damage occurred in the B-6 level that houses the PATH train station. Other emerging issues that complicated the rescue efforts were that reportedly 1.8 million gallons of water had collected in the sub-basement levels from ruptured pipes and would need to be pumped out, and the presence of asbestos throughout the building in areas that had yet to undergo the abatement process.

Within hours of the blast, over fifty groups had telephoned authorities to claim responsibility for the terrorist bombing. We would learn, as it was confirmed several days later, that an Islamic extremist group, allegedly headed by Sheik Omar Abdul Rahman, was responsible for this heinous crime. Three members of the group, Mohammed Salameh, Nidal Ayyad, and Mahmud Abouhalima, have since been arrested by the FBI and NYPD and charged with various crimes associated with the World Trade Center bombing. U.S. and international law enforcement officials continue the investigation and pursuit of others who might have participated. A note of interest in this case is that "Sheik Omar Abdul Rahman, a fundamentalist extremist who hates Western values and is an avowed enemy of the United States, Israel, and the notions of secular governments in the Islamic world, has been tied to the assassinations of Egyptian President Anwar el-Sadat and Rabbi Meir Kahane (founder of the Jewish Defense League), as well as to other acts of violence both in Egypt and in the United States." (*The New York Post,* "The Reality of Terrorism," March 9, 1993.) In the Sadat incident, Rahman was acquitted for lack of evidence, and he was never charged in the Kahane murder. "The suspects appear to be tied spiritually to Rahman…Before arriving here, Sheik Omar was better known as the man who issued the fatwa (religious orders) calling for the assassination of Anwar Sadat. Some 107 of his followers were convicted for their roles in the uprising surrounding that killing." (*The New York Post*, "The Reality of Terrorism," March 9, 1993.)

Structuring and Managing the Incident

Upon arrival I conducted a face-to-face meeting with Lts. Torres, Browne, and Fenton, and Capts. Armstrong and Olsen to begin implementation of the EMS Incident Management System (IMS). Capt. Armstrong was designated the Safety Officer, Capt. Olsen was assigned to assess the situation in One WTC, Lt. Browne was to assess the Winter Garden Theater, Lt. Torres was to assess the Triage Sector for One WTC, and Lt. Fenton was to assess Two World Trade Center.

The EMS IMS is clearly delineated within the *NYC*EMS Operating Guide* under our Emergency Medical Action Plan (EMAP). It is the constant use of IMS at each and every incident to which NYC*EMS responds that permitted the fluid management of this massive incident, and it is one of the crucial reasons that this incident was managed with success. All members of NYC*EMS undergo training with the EMS IMS, from trainees in the academy right on up to ranking officers.

As I assumed command of the signal 10-30 (Explosion), the initial incident presented us with a myriad of complex issues: thick acrid smoke pouring from the West Street entrance ramps to the underground parking facility and the WTC Towers, numerous people evacuating the affected buildings throughout the WTC campus and seeking EMS assistance, thick shards of glass raining down on the civilians and rescuers from One World Trade Center and the Vista Hotel, and the inclement weather elements of snow, ice, and rain.

After receiving the initial updates from each of the officers detailed to assess proximal locations to the blast area, it was determined that at least three divisions would be needed to effectively manage this incident. These divisions were: One WTC Operations under the command of D/C Edward Gabriel, Vista Hotel Operations under the command of Captain Robert Iannarelli, and Two WTC Operations under the command of D/C Michael Rice. As each operational division was implemented, the requisite sectors were also established to support those operations, i.e., triage, treatment, and transport. This would permit the necessary allocation of resources, allowing for tracking of units, personnel, and patients in each specific area as best as possible considering the huge scope of the event.

A central staging sector was established at West Street and Vesey Street, with Lt. John Perruggia as the Sector Officer to coordinate and control all vehicle/unit distribution. In addition, Capt. Joseph Apuzzo, Lt. Richard Garcia, and Lt. Steven Sammis were detailed to be the control/access officers to keep units from being pulled into the site unnecessarily and to limit freelancing of units. This strategy was extremely effective, providing us with greater accountability of the units that were requested into the site from Staging and a passport system to track unit movement in and out of the incident site. I cannot overemphasize the importance that these roles played in the management of resources. Another key asset was the utilization of the EMS Field Communications Unit. Upon the arrival of this unit, D/C James Basile assumed the responsibility for coordinating communications from the incident site as the Communications Sector Officer.

Shortly after the primary deployment of resources, Lt. Browne reported back to me that he had an estimated 200 patients in the Winter Garden Theater who would require assessment and possible treatment. The creation of a fourth division, Winter Garden Operations, under the command of Lt. Robert Browne, was now necessary to better manage this area.

Early in the incident, several strategic requests would prove to help maintain operations at the incident site as well as assist with the maintenance of normal 9-1-1 responses. First, with the response of senior EMS management to the site, I had immediate access to Chief David L. Diggs, NYC*EMS Executive Director; Mr. Vincent Clark, Deputy Executive Director; Dr. Lorraine Giordano, Medical Director; Chief MacNeil C. Cross, Chief of Operations; and Ms. Lynn Schulman, Associate Executive Director for Public Information. On-site access to these officials permitted quick implementation of decisions regarding issues such as holding over an entire NYC*EMS tour from the day shift and redeployment of members of the service in reserve ambulances to support the citywide operation, as well as the transportation of spare members to the site for relief purposes. The canceling of training classes at the EMS Academy and redeployment of members to the site also proved beneficial. Activation of the NYC*EMS Mutual Aid Radio System (MARS) helped to muster assistance from the volunteer ambulance corps within NYC. An unprecedented formal request for mutual aid from units in New Jersey and from commercial ambulances in New York City proved to be key in the overall success of the operation.

A/C Pedro Carrasquillo was assigned to the role of Liaison Officer to help expedite requests for interagency assistance to support the EMS operation. Chiefs Walter Drivet and Keith McCabe of University of Medicine and Dentistry of New Jersey EMS arrived at the scene and were immediately assigned to coordinate the New Jersey mutual aid resources that were responding to the incident. Upon the arrival of a field communications unit from the Ridgefield Park, New Jersey First Aid Squad, we were able to position this unit parallel to the NYC*EMS Field Communications, coordinating New Jersey unit access and movement to and from the site. In addition, Chief Joseph Cali of Jersey City Medical Center EMS established a staging location on the New Jersey side of the Holland Tunnel for all NYC-bound units. This permitted the resources to be organized into task forces that could be escorted to the incident site as they were needed.

Expanded Operations

As incident operations continued, the need to redeploy arriving resources to other areas to support the ever-growing patient numbers became evident. A/C Zachary

Goldfarb was assigned to assume responsibility for Two WTC operations and D/C Rice for coordinating interior operations at Two WTC. As the numbers of patients continued to rise in the previously established divisions, repeated calls for EMS were being received at two additional locations. Upon assessment of conditions on the Vesey Street side of the WTC, it was determined that another division would be required. Capt. Michael Garufi assumed responsibility for the Vesey Street Operations. At the same time, Capt. Andrew Tychnowitz reported that numerous patients had congregated at the Five WTC site and were in need of EMS assistance. Capt. Tychnowitz was assigned as the Five WTC Operations Officer.

One of the more effective tactics that was employed at the division level was a forward triage station located on the upper floors of the towers. In each instance as victims were being evacuated through darkened, smoke-filled stairwells, EMS crews were enabled to conduct a cursory triage. In an incident of this origin and magnitude, one would expect trauma to be the prevalent injury. This was not the case. We experienced numerous minor trauma patients, but the overwhelming number of patients were those with smoke inhalation, exhaustion, and aggravation of pre-existing medical conditions, i.e., C.O.P.D., asthma, cardiac, hypertensive crisis, etc. Also encountered at the site was a high number of pregnant patients who had been exposed to the above-listed elements.

Another tactic employed that assisted greatly was the utilization of transit buses with EMS personnel and equipment on them and police escorts to transport numerous patients with minor injuries to area hospitals. This permitted us to conserve the use of ambulances for the more serious patients requiring transport to designated hospitals.

Another element that was handled through the coordination of the Field Communications and EMS Communications Divisions was monitoring the available bed status in New York City and surrounding communities. In addition to the standard bed status, the availability of trauma, burn, and hyperbaric beds was assessed frequently to avoid overloading any one facility. This information was provided to the EMS Incident Commander and Division Transport Officers to guide transportation destination decisions.

Consistent with the growing numbers of patients and the anticipated extended operations, the development of several other support sectors was imperative to ensure the effectiveness of overall incident management.

With a significant media presence on-site, the need for a public information liaison is self-explanatory. Under the direction of Ms. Schulman (AED/Public Information), a public information sector was established. EMTs Sandra Mackay and Robert Leonard helped to balance the plethoric demands for information and access to EMS operations and officers on-site. At EMS headquarters, Inspector Charles DeGaetano provided support by managing the non-stop telephone inquiries for information and updates.

Assessment of long-term needs regarding the maintenance of normal 9-1-1 operations and those associated with the WTC incident was of significant importance. Chief MacNeil Cross, Chief of Operations, requested that this assignment be given a high priority. Based upon the fact that the incident was in Manhattan, the task was assigned to A/C Pedro Carrasquillo, Manhattan Borough Commander. With the assistance of D/C Steven Kuhr, fundamental strategies were developed to conduct on-site relief and assignment of units to provide WTC coverage for the 12 hours after the "acute" event had been secured so that we could assume a long-term operation posture. This area was designated as the planning sector. A/C Ulysses Grant replaced A/C Carrasquillo as the Liaison Sector Officer at the Interagency Command Post.

Earlier in the incident, D/C Jerry Gombo had activated the NYC*EMS Emergency Operations Center at EMS headquarters. At this location the coordination of all EMS resources—with the goal of maintenance of full system effectiveness—took place. This difficult task was accomplished with the assistance of the staff from the Office of the Chief of Operations (OCO) and Chief John Lazzaro, D/C Mark Steffens, and D/C Thomas Ryan of the Communications Division. These individuals were confronted with a relentless task that became very complicated at times. What needs to be understood is that, as unbelievable as this might sound, the World Trade Center incident was only one of over 3,100 calls for help that the NYC*EMS system would be called upon to respond to on this date. Constant juggling and redeployment of available resources would need to be accomplished over a twelve-hour period in order to ensure proper response to all who requested EMS assistance. Additionally, OCO was required to send a representative to the NYC Mayor's Office of Emergency Management, Command and Control Center, to help with the overall citywide impact coordination and the role that NYC*EMS would need to provide.

Consistent with the highly specialized operations that were being conducted on-site, and in addition to the roles already mentioned in which the NYC*EMS Special Operations Division (SOD) was engaged, there existed the need for several other sectors. The utilization of NYPD aviation helicopters to evacuate patients through the airlifting of rescuers to the roofs of the World Trade Center Towers necessitated the establishment of a Med E Vac Operations Sector. Lt. Roy David of SOD was assigned this task. Lt. Kevin Haugh of SOD was assigned to the SOD tactical support sector. With the assistance of the Emergency Response Squad, a group of highly trained EMTs in SOD, all support functions were executed, from electrical power supply and scene lighting to being poised to conduct hazardous materials decontamination in the event it became necessary (the latter under the direction of Lt. JoAnn Mack as the Haz Mat Sector Officer).

In order to maintain an adequate supply of equipment at the incident, five logistical support units and two Quartermaster Response Trucks responded to the site, and a formal logistics sector was established under the direction of Capt. Jace Pinkus. In addition to ensuring access and distribution of the supplies, Capt. Pinkus was also required to institute a system for tracking and recovery of equipment that was issued.

Ensuring the physical and mental health needs of rescuers at an incident of this magnitude is no small task. Capt. Fran Pascale was assigned to establish the rehab sector. By using NYC MTA transit buses for shelter, the EMS members of the service were afforded a rest area temporarily away from the elements of the weather and the demands of the scene. Food was available through the generosity of the American Red Cross, Salvation Army, and cafeteria facilities of Merrill Lynch and American Express. I extend my sincere thanks and appreciation to these organizations for their assistance and generosity to all the rescuers. All too often the care givers forget to give themselves or their brothers and sisters care at these incidents. Thankfully this was not the case at the WTC incident. On the mental health side, the NYC*EMS CISD team was activated and under the supervision of Ms. Lori Sullivan and Ms. Susan Sabor. On-site evaluations, assistance, and long-term evaluation strategies were quickly developed to aid all EMS MOS.

The final sector that was established was a morgue sector. This area received four of the five DOAs that were recovered that day. The fifth DOA was pronounced at the hospital after a unit transported him as a traumatic arrest. At this location the proper tracking and identification documentation was completed and a constant interface with officials from various agencies (PAPD, NYPD, FBI, and Chief Medical Examiner's Office) took place. Eventually the bodies were transported to the Chief Medical Examiner's Officer for further forensic investigation. The sixth DOA would be recovered weeks later.

Securement of the "Acute" Event

More than twelve-and-a-half hours into the incident the scene was secured, with more than 1,043 patients generated by the bombing of the World Trade Center. Of these numbers, 632 patients had EMS contact, 450 of whom were transported to 17 hospitals in three boroughs. A total of 176 were treated and released on the scene and six deaths were attributed to the event. The aggregate of patients above the 632 sought treatment at hospitals on their own.

The decision to secure the scene was made in order to start the incident reconstruction activities for the "acute" event and capture all associated activities for the WTC bombing on a single NYC*EMS Computer Aided Dispatch (CAD) call number. "Acute event" is defined as the activities and injuries that immediately surrounded the bombing itself. The long-term activities would encompass a separate accounting and reconstruction process, utilizing separate CAD numbers each day the operation was in existence.

Long-Term Operations and Support

After numerous on-site interagency meetings throughout the day, it was quickly determined that Operations would need to make the transition from reactionary to extended. The initial reports by the Port Authority of New York and New Jersey structural engineers was that it would be at least several weeks before they could complete shoring operations. The primary concern was for the B-5 level, which was presently supporting the rubble of the blast and the fear of secondary collapses. The blast produced damage that created almost 2,700 cubic tons of debris that would need removal from the sub-grade level. This activity would be an ongoing process while the search teams and investigators operated in the area termed "ground zero," the epicenter of the blast.

In order to properly support EMS operations during this stage of the incident, a request to activate the NYC*EMS collapse medic component of the NYC Interagency FEMA USAR Team was made and approved. Although this program is still in its implementation phase, I was able to access members of the service who had previously volunteered to participate in this program. In most cases they already had some training in operating in this type of environment and would be able to quickly interface with the other rescue workers, should a secondary collapse occur and rescuers become injured or trapped. By temporarily reassigning these members from their present commands to the WTC detail, we were able to decrease some of the mounting costs of the operation.

Although we initially operated under the pretense that there was only one person unaccounted for, the prevailing feeling among most rescuers was, if that was truly the case, we were very lucky. The day of the blast was wet, snowy, and windy. Based upon the weather, even if there was no one else present in the garage blast area at the time (lunch time) of the explosion, the possibility of homeless people seeking refuge from the elements was a plausible concern. We would later find out that, although we had valid fears, they were unfounded, with the last missing victim of the blast being recovered on the B-5 level under several feet of rubble seventeen days after the explosion. The consensus of all parties involved was that we were extremely fortunate that we were not forced to confront a greater number of trapped patients.

More immediate concerns that emerged were the logistical issues that surround an extended operation such as this. Through the courtesy of the Port Authority of New York and New Jersey, the owners of the WTC Complex, a 10 ft. × 40 ft. trailer was brought to the site for use as an EMS temporary headquarters vehicle (THV). In order to enhance the effectiveness of the extended operations, the following equipment was requested and brought to the scene: EMS Radio Services delivered a full radio complement including 400 MHz and 800 MHz bases, portable radio rack chargers, and spare batteries installed in the trailer; EMS Information Technology Division delivered a 486 computer and laser printer with full software support and a CAD dispatch terminal and modem permitting us to compartmentalize the operation, control the dispatch and assignment of units on-site, and support the lower Manhattan 9-1-1 operation because of the impact that traffic closures in the area were having on travel times; Consolidated Edison provided full power to the trailer; New York Telephone provided on request five voice lines and three data lines; and Bell South Communication Systems provided all the telephone instruments and a facsimile machine necessary to ensure the consistency of the EMS continued operations.

The EMS resources that were assigned to the extended WTC detail consisted of:

One (1)   Chief Officer Tour 2 and 3
One (1)   Captain All Tours

Two (2)   Lieutenants 1 - Staging/Triage; 1 - Safety Officer [SOD]
One (1)   Dispatcher
Two (2)   ALS Units 1 - On-site; 1 - Collapse Medic Unit
Two (2)   BLS Units 1 - On-site; 1 - Haz/Tac
One (1)   SOD Emergency Response Squad

Implementation of twelve-hour tours instead of the standard eight proved to be beneficial to both EMS and to the members who would be operating at the incident. The utilization of these resources were assessed on a daily and weekly basis in meetings that were held between Chief Robert McCracken, Chief of Field Services, and myself. Our meetings were convened after the two daily on-site interagency meetings. Risk assessment, structural stability, call volume, patients generated at the site, and the numbers of people operating in the "hole" were taken into consideration.

While we were still operating at this incident and at the over 3,000 calls a day we normally respond to, the City of New York was hit with the worst blizzard of the decade. The winds at the WTC site were clocked at 78.4 mph at one point, and required us to install additional shoring to the EMS THV because of the potential for it shifting and/or flipping over. Additional safety precautions were taken with EMS vehicle positioning and taping of windows for fear of breaking glass. After the storm passed, another safety concern arose from large chunks of ice, some as large as 6 ft. long, 3 ft. wide and 3 in. thick, that were falling off the towers and causing damage to vehicles, surrounding structures, and a high hazard to public safety personnel working in the area. Constant monitoring of this condition and declaring a hard-hat (helmets worn) operation was necessary until the Port Authority maintenance personnel were able to mitigate this condition.

Further considerations that were addressed included the ability to feed the EMS members of the service who were assigned to the extended operation and unable to leave the scene to procure meals. This concern was not unique to NYC*EMS but was shared by the multitudes of agencies that were operating on the scene. The Port Authority secured a location within One World Trade Center to serve food six times a day. The "disaster diner," as it was dubbed, provided a small haven for my members and gave them a break from the rigors of this scene, along with the opportunity to meet with other rescuers and officials who were operating at the incident.

The presence of U.S. Department of Labor, Occupational Health and Safety and the N.Y.S. Public Employee Safety Health Officers provided some interesting issues for all agencies to address on scene. First, all members were closely scrutinized for proper personal protective equipment and its applications. Next, a decision was made that all personnel who could operate in the sub-grade levels would be required to undergo pulmonary function tests, be fit-tested, and taught the use of APRs because of the dust levels and the potential of asbestos. This had little effect on the members of EMS SOD because of the stringent medical standards that they must adhere to during the Haz Mat physical assessment process, but it did require us to have the officers and line units assigned to the detail complete this process prior to going on-site. The testing process and equipment was provided, once again, by the Port Authority.

Because of the need to enhance security and limit access to the affected sixteen-acre campus, all persons, regardless of whether in uniform or not, were required to secure credentials for access to the site. These credentials, similar to concert backstage passes, established what level of access clearance an individual was granted. EMS personnel who were assigned to the incident for the long term were issued All Area Access, while the transient overtime units were given escorts to areas when required. Due to the crime scene and the ongoing investigation, access to the area was kept to an "as required" basis.

As the risks lessened, the level of EMS presence was gradually decreased, until the operation was finally secured on 3/20/93 Tour 2, with over 90 more patients being treated by EMS at the WTC site. The decision to secure the EMS operation was based upon the site becoming a "pure" reconstruction site, rather then a rescue/recovery/crime scene.

Summary

In retrospect, I find that some extraordinary tasks were accomplished by extraordinary people. To the members of New York City Emergency Medical Service, Volunteer Ambulance Corps of NYC, the New Jersey Mutual Units, and the commercial ambulance personnel who jumped in to assist with this unprecedented event, I salute you and thank you for your dedication and commitment to pre-hospital care.

Down the line we have learned many lessons that will be shared with the profession and future generations of EMTs and paramedics to come. Many of these lessons will be incorporated immediately in the way we respond to mass casualty incidents and disasters. We were confronted with a monumental challenge, never faced before in the history of the New York City Emergency Medical Service, and we were able to effectively respond to it consistent with the highest traditions of Emergency Medical Services. This incident is truly a story of teamwork, because, without it, many more people would have been injured or possibly died. To the hundreds of EMS professionals who responded, all I can say is, I'm proud to call you my peers and extend my heartfelt thanks for your assistance.

APPENDIX I
ADDITIONAL ACCOUNTS OF
EMS INCIDENT MANAGEMENT IN
THE REAL WORLD

"When the Mighty Mississippi Lived Up To Its Name," by Gary Ludwig
"On the Job in Colonial Heights, Virginia," by Dennis L. Rubin
"High-rise Fire in Wilmington, Delware," by Lawrence Tan
"Incident in Westwood, California," by James P. Denney
"The AmTrak Sunset Limited Disaster in Mobile, Alabama," by Paul R. Smith
"I-10 Bayway Accident in Mobile, Alabama," by Paul R. Smith

WHEN THE MIGHTY MISSISSIPPI LIVED UP TO ITS NAME

By Gary G. Ludwig, MS, EMT-P, Chief Paramedic, St. Louis Fire Department, St. Louis, MO

> I do not know much about gods, but I think that the river is a strong brown god—sullen, untamed and intractable. Patient to some degree, at first recognized as a frontier; useful, untrustworthy, as a conveyer of commerce; Then only a problem confronting the builder of bridges. The problem once solved, the brown god is almost forgotten by the dwellers in the cities—ever, however, implacable, keeping his seasons and rages, unpropitiated by worshipers of the machine, but waiting, watching and waiting.
>
> T.S. Elliott, *The Dry Salvages*

The Mississippi River, 2,348 miles long, is the second longest river, after the Missouri River, in the United States. Unfortunately for St. Louis, both rivers meet in a confluence with the Illinois River just north of the city of St. Louis, before flowing by the Gateway Arch. The Mississippi River provides a drainage area for about 40% of the country, and runs through or touches all or part of 31 states in the west. The Mississippi is a friend to many with irrigation for crops, transportation of commerce by barge from city to city, and provision of recreation. Because of unusually heavy rains in the upper midwest during the months of April and May of 1993, the Mississippi River became a foe to many who depend upon it. The first warning for St. Louis was on June 25, 1993, when the Army Corps of Engineers warned that rain in the north would cause substantial flooding in St. Louis. By June 27th the river rose above what is considered the flood stage mark of 30 feet.

St. Louis, approximately 63 square miles, is a port city on the Mississippi River. The city of St. Louis is a county within itself, with its eastern border the Mississippi River. The population in St. Louis is approximately 400,000, but it swells to approximately one million during the business day.

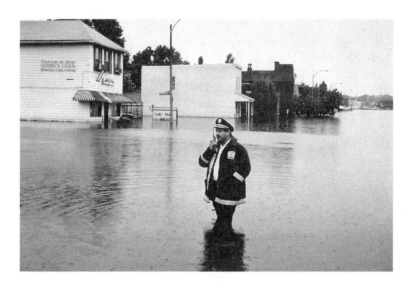

Emergency medical services and all 9-1-1 medical calls are handled by St. Louis EMS, a "third service" operation. (The operation is now a part of the St. Louis Fire Department.) Consisting of some 172 personnel, the system handles roughly 65,000 emergency calls a year. St. Louis EMS has a fleet of 30 ambulances, numerous support and administrative vehicles, including a 42-seat-passenger bus that was converted into a mobile command post.

In July and August of 1993 the Emergency Medical Service for the city of St. Louis was tested in not only resources, but manpower and fortitude. Unlike most disasters, floods lend themselves to prediction and precision. Tornadoes skip and veer, hurricanes seem to wallow at whim, and large fires with multiple patients can come and go before you can even get to the scene. But a flood has only one way to go, and it usually follows a schedule. Each morning the 0800 staff meeting, which consisted of managers of the involved city, federal, and private agencies would meet in the Emergency Operations Center of the City's Emergency Management Agency (CEMA). Each meeting would include a report from each agency, including the Army of Corps of Engineers. The Army Corps of Engineers would start off with a report from the hydrologist. Hand a hydrologist a contour map and form numbers on upstream rainfall and river readings, and you'll get back with great accuracy figures on which basements and streets will go under water and when.

The trouble is that this year's numbers refused to sit still. Upriver from St. Louis, the rain kept falling and the rivers kept rising. The longer the rain continued, the longer water-soaked levees strained to hold back the water. Eventually many levees broke and flooded farmlands, destroying 1993 crops. St. Louis is not farmland. It is a densely populated urban city, whose economy and residents are protected by a flood wall running for an 11-mile stretch adjacent to most parts of the city's waterfront. The rest of the city's riverfront is protected by high bluffs and earthen levees. However, some areas are unprotected. One area that particularly plagued emergency personnel in St. Louis was the River des Peres. River des Peres is a watershed basin that conveys most storm water from the central part of St. Louis County, through the south part of the city, finally emptying in the Mississippi River. The problem was not storm water, but backup of river water from the Mississippi River. As the Mississippi rose, so did the River des Peres. The flood stage in St. Louis is at the 30-foot mark. As of this writing, the river has crested three times, with the highest crest being at 49.4 feet on August 3rd, 19.4 feet over flood stage. In parts of the country, the Mississippi River was described as 8–10 miles out of its banks.

Mitigation

The first stage of any disaster is the mitigation stage. EMS providers are generally not involved in the mitigation phase of a flood disaster. In mitigation, the attempt should be made to control or reduce the disaster, long before the emergency occurs. A prime example of this was the construction of the flood wall on the St. Louis riverfront. The flood was designed to handle a flood up to the 54-foot mark. Unfortunately, it became apparent that the force and power of water can overcome anything manmade. Flood gates were closed along the wall to provide a continuous wall. The second month of the flood emergency, St. Louis officials were concerned about possible breaches in the levee wall. Breaches can occur not only at the flood gates, but under the wall, as well. On July 23 a 20-foot hole was created on the dry pavement side of the flood wall when water forced a path under a 24-foot wide, six-foot-deep footing of concrete supporting the flood wall. If a breach of any of the gates or wall were to occur at the highest point of the flood, which was 49.4 feet, an entire, densely populated, commercial and residential area stretching some 8 miles long and 1 mile wide would have been saturated with water.

Preparedness

The first warnings from the Army Corps of Engineers triggered the City's Emergency Management Agency (CEMA) into action. Often disasters will occur regardless of the efficiency of mitigation efforts. The preparedness phase of any disaster involves putting actions and plans into play that would minimize the impact of a disaster. The optimum preparedness phase involves planning for the most efficient and effective response to minimize injury and loss of life. The preparedness phase involved all vital city agencies meeting to develop a plan of attack if flooding were to occur. This involved looking at contour maps to determine what would be flooded at the 40-foot level versus the 48-foot level. Early in the planning stages, officials had no idea that water would reach the magnitude of the 49.4-foot mark. It was determined that the 43-foot mark would be the key indicator for the response phase of city agencies.

   The preparedness phase for St. Louis EMS involved the establishment of staging areas, a check of resources and supplies, rescheduling employees to optimize human resources, and coordination with other city agencies responsible for the response phase of the flooding disaster. On July 11, the Army Corps of Engineers notified the city of St. Louis that on July 16 the flood stage along the River des Peres would reach the 43-foot mark. It was at this point that the city agencies switched from a preparedness phase into the response phase.

Response

The response phase of this flooding disaster was a prolonged and challenging chain of events that would test the St. Louis EMS system repeatedly with one misfortune after another. Up to the time of this writing, the St. Louis EMS system was tested with three record crests, levee breaks, one optional evacuation, two mandatory evacuations, sudden and severe thunderstorms with flash flooding, tornadoes, two fires in a propane tank farm, three break-away riverboat attractions on the St. Louis riverfront, and dignitary visits.

   As with any disaster, each agency plays a vital role in supporting a disaster operation. In St. Louis, EMS supported the flood operations in a variety of ways. One of the first decisions in the preparedness phase was the establishment of a forward command post for police, fire, and EMS, near the flood-affected areas. Carondelet Park, a large city park, was chosen for the established command site. The site provided an opportunity to keep curiosity seekers and press away, while still providing easy access to the flood-affected areas. A press center was established near the command post, in order to allow senior staff to field press inquiries in the vicinity of the affected flood area.

The establishment of any EMS command post for a long-term operation in St. Louis involves activating the EMS mobile command post. The mobile command post is a converted 42-passenger bus donated to EMS by the public transportation authority for the St. Louis area. Conversion included painting and decaling the outside of the bus, removal of some seats, and the installation of workstations and tables with radios and computers for communications with all city agencies, plus fire/EMS districts in St. Louis County. Once on site, telephone lines were installed for voice and data communications. Computers were hooked up and connected directly to the CAD system at the EMS communications center for instantaneous information pertaining to street unit availability, as well as to the disaster. The computers' fax capability allowed reports to be generated on site to be immediately faxed into the Emergency Operations Center of CEMA. The fax capability was also important for receiving instantaneous information from a contracted weather service, which would fax hourly updates on weather reports for the south St. Louis area. In several cases, the unstable air over the midwest suddenly produced violent thunderstorms and flash flooding near the flood-affected areas. Flash flooding occurred several times over the course of the two-month operation, and on July 31 tornado warnings were issued for the city of St. Louis when multiple tornadoes were spotted aloft throughout the metropolitan area.

Sudden and violent thunderstorms can and did produce over 2–4 inches of rain within an hour. The effect of flash flooding played havoc on the levee walls. During and after the storm, levee walls gave way and caused immediate flooding of the nearby areas. The electric utility company provided a power drop to the bus, and tied it into a circuit breaker box already configured on the bus. A large air conditioner was then powered, providing the cooling necessary for St. Louis summers, while still providing power for lights, radios, and computer equipment. Also staged at the command post site was St. Louis EMS's disaster response vehicle (DRV). The DRV is a converted ambulance whose interior has been removed and replaced with metal shelving. Inside this vehicle is all required equipment for dealing with any multicasualty event, such as 25 backboards, 14 jump kits, and multi-port oxygen tanks.

Once the command post was established, a detailed map was drawn of the flood-affected areas. The most flood-prone areas in south St. Louis included over 1,500 homes and businesses, running some three miles back from the mouth of where the River des Peres empties into the Mississippi. Contour maps provided by the sewer district gave indications of what would flood at different river stage levels. The detailed map was divided into sectors based on geography and ease of access. As the situation deteriorated, the entire St. Louis riverfront from one end of the city to the other was divided into labeled sectors and preplanned with staging areas and command posts in the event one of the flood gates or levee walls gave way.

Early in the response phase of the flooding emergency, the Office of Public Safety for the city of St. Louis initiated an evacuation and cut power and gas to those homes and businesses that were located in the contours of the flood-prone areas. The evacuation was optional. Many people chose to stay without electricity and gas. One of the many roles that EMS played was to perform daily checks on residents on a "critical list." This list was developed with the help of the power utility company and a door-to-door survey of residents in the area. Residents on this "critical list" were people whose lives were dependent upon electricity or had some type of medical condition that might be aggravated by the lack of electricity. The survey and medical list produced people who were on home ventilators, used electric wheel chairs, and had a multitude of other medical conditions. Each day St. Louis paramedics would visit the homes of these people to check on their current condition and determine if any further assistance would be required from the city. In some cases, the residents were evaluated and taken to the hospital when it was determined that their health was deteriorating. EMS paramedics also assisted disabled individuals who chose to evacuate to a friend or relative's home. At times an ambulance was required, but on most occasions, a specially equipped van, working under the auspices of a St. Louis service that cared for disabled people was utilized.

Sandbagging Operations

One of the most critical operations of the flooding was to raise the levees with sandbags. A request for volunteers was disseminated by the St. Louis Streets and Forestry Departments three weekends in succession resulted in a phenomenal response. As the rivers would rise, the levee walls would have to go higher. Volunteers were asked to report to a staging area several miles away from the sandbagging operations. From there they were bused into the sandbag production site or to the levee where sandbags were needed. On any given day, there were approximately 2,000–2,500 people sandbagging. Sandbagging operations were hampered by the typical St. Louis weather in July and August with its high heat and humidity. Heat indexes (the combination of heat and humidity to produce what the temperature really feels like) went well over 100 degrees on several days, prompting the St. Louis Health Department to issue heat alerts.

One of EMS's most important roles was to support the sandbagging by providing heat relief and minor first aid to the volunteer sandbaggers. The heat relief was the primary concern. At each sandbagging site, EMS crews established cooling stations on large passenger buses and provided icewater-soaked towels. Water sprays were set up by the St. Louis Fire Department, and the Red Cross and Salvation Army provided cool drinks and food. Paramedics patrolled the sandbagging operations, looking for volunteers who might be yielding to the heat. Band-aids and aspirin would be used during the entire operation. In all, six volunteers were transported to the hospital suffering from heat exhaustion.

Levee Breaks

At any given time, and at any place, a water-soaked earthen and sandbag levee could and did break. Immediately, all EMS crews assigned to the flood detail were told to report to a level-one staging area near the incident. Four additional paramedic units and a field supervisor redirected from street operations were also dispatched to a level-two staging area at the command post in Carondelet Park. After conferring with the sewer district officials and reviewing the contoured maps, it would be immediately known what area would flood. Paramedics would converge on what would be the affected areas to notify any residents, who had not voluntarily evacuated, to evacuate immediately due to the impending rushing water. Sometimes this was done on foot, if time allowed. Other times, PA systems on the ambulance were used to make the notifications. Other paramedic crews from the level-two staging area would support Street and Forestry Department crews who would converge on the breach with strike teams of front end loaders and over 50 loaded dump trucks of sandbags. Working in rushing water up to their chests was extremely dangerous. In many cases, the breach would be "plugged," but on several occasions strike teams and EMS crews were pulled out because the water level was just too unsafe. These areas, along with the homes and businesses, would be completely inundated with water within a short period of time. Another danger to the flood emergency was "sand boils." Sand boils are areas on the dry side of the levee walls that are saturated with water underground. The water attempts to force its way up out of the ground to equalize with the water on the flooded side of the levee walls. In some cases, it was not uncommon to see a city street rise three feet in the course of ten minutes.

A PIVOTAL TIME

The days of July 30, 31, August 1 and 2 would become a true test of the St. Louis EMS system. On July 30 a flooded Phillips Petroleum propane tank farm, near where the River des Peres empties into the Mississippi, reached a critical point. A total of 51 tanks, each containing 30,000 gallons of liquified propane, began shifting and floating in the flooded waters. As the tanks began to float and shift, stress was placed on the valves under each tank. Leaks were detected, prompting St. Louis officials and Phillips Petroleum personnel to make decisions on how to resolve this critical situation. While experts were flying in from all parts of the nation to help remedy the situation, the determination was made to initiate a mandatory evacuation of a half-mile radius of the tank farm. On July 30th that evacuation took place. St. Louis police and firefighters went door-to-door notifying residents. St. Louis EMS set up a forward command post in the back of the deputy chief's van in the affected area utilizing the incident command structure. This command post was known as "Boniface Command," since the command post was established in a small park outside the St. Boniface Catholic Church. A staging area was established with ambulances, transportation buses, and specifically equipped vans for the disabled in another part of the affected area. As a request would be received for someone who required medical evaluation or was in need of special assistance, a triage officer was sent to the scene to evaluate the needs of the individual. The triage officer would then contact the staging officer and request manpower and equipment.

After evaluation by the experts, the decision was made to slowly bleed the tanks, creating a slow release of propane into the air with eventual dissipation. All ignition sources were eliminated because all electric and gas was cut within the half-mile affected evacuation area. On August 1 at around 7 p.m., the radios at the Carondelet Park command post began cracking that there was a flash fire in the propane tank farm and one of the tanks was on fire. Immediately, all EMS crews in the flood affected area were told to report to the level-two staging area, with additional crews and field supervisors dispatched to support the operation. The level-two staging area was in the cold zone, since it pertains to a hazardous material incident. A roll call of bed availability was immediately initiated by the St. Louis EMS communications center over a computerized network. Two alarms were struck by the St. Louis Fire Department to supplement their already established task force for the propane tank farm operation. The fire was extinguished, but not without extensive damage to a one-story brick building on the propane tank farm. Evidently vapor from the propane found an ignition source, creating the fire. As of this writing, the source of the ignition has not been determined. Five tanks containing eight-inch pipes were of particular concern. Computer modeling and further evaluation showed a release of all five simultaneously would produce a 4000 ft. × 4000 ft., twelve-foot-high cloud of propane gas.

With the new computer model predictions, the half-mile radius was not sufficient. Therefore, the decision was made to expand the mandatory evacuation area to a one-mile radius. Starting at 6 a.m. on August 2, the evacuation of 1,300 homes and 11,800 people began. EMS would play the same role as before, providing assistance to those infirmed and to those individuals with medical needs. Since the area was larger than the first evacuation, three sectors were set up. These sectors corresponded with the maps already sectored when the command post was established. Each sector was assigned a field supervisor. Hence, under the incident command system, call letters were known as "Sector G, H, or I Command." A staging area was established outside the affected area with ambulances, buses, and specialty vans for the disabled. The command post in Carondelet Park coordinated the evacuation. A major challenge of the evacuation was moving the residents of a nursing home. Within three hours, the entire evacuation was completed.

The propane tank quandary has yet to be resolved. In the history of the United States, no incident of this type has ever been encountered. Officials of Phillips Petroleum told the media, "We are writing the book on this one." In preparation for any cataclysmic event, an explosion at the propane tank farm was pre-planned. Staging areas for ambulances from other EMS/fire districts were established, and treatment sites for the injured were organized in a cold zone outside the one-mile radius. Medical equipment, along with multi-casualty provisions were pre-staged for days in the treatment area in the event something tragic were to occur.

Hazardous Materials

With the rise of the river, many commercial and industrial complexes besides the propane tank farm were affected. It was not uncommon to see railroad tank cars and large chemical holding tanks sitting in water. On one particular site, holding tanks containing 750,000 gallons of benzene were submerged in river water. At another site, a railroad tank car containing PCBs was completely submerged. In preparation for any major release that might occur, all sites were pre-planned in regard to what type of chemical(s) was on-site, what the health hazards would be, and the necessary treatment if contact was made with the product by rescue personnel or civilians. All information was logged into computers in the command post, and, if necessary, could be instantly recalled and printed out by sector.

Recovery

The fourth stage of any disaster is recovery. The recovery phase of any flood emergency can be just as intensive and far-reaching as the response phase. Besides the health hazards of mosquitos and contamination of the water from chemicals, the prospects are great for someone cleaning a flooded home to encounter river snakes, rats, and leeches. Part of the recovery phase for St. Louis EMS included employees who worked the flood detail to be debriefed by critical incident stress debriefing teams. The concern for the employees relates to the stress of working long periods without rest and little time off. Although briefings were available during the flood emergency, employees were encouraged, once the flood waters had receded, to take advantage of this service.

Stretching Resources

Unlike a fire, plane crash, or train accident, floods are not quite so dramatic. However, high-intensity scenarios, as previously mentioned, are of much shorter duration than the flood experienced in St. Louis in 1993. Of particular concern to the administration of St. Louis EMS were fatigue factors of personnel and the stretching of resources over prolonged periods of time. Overtime personnel were necessary to maintain the staffing levels needed for the flood operations. EMS crews assigned to the flood emergency were often held over based upon the predictions of the river stage. During prolonged flooding, rivers tend to lower and rise. The Mississippi River in St. Louis has crested three times. In other words, the river has gone down, but then rose again to a new height due to rainfall from the north. Therefore, the need to have the maximum amount of personnel assigned to the emergency was not as significant when the river stage lowered. Minimum staffing was necessary for the maintenance of assignments required to be performed by EMS. Usually one week ahead of time, EMS administration knew if flooding or levees would break based upon predictions made by the Army Corps of Engineers. It was at these critical times that additional EMS crews were placed on duty for the flood emergency. Sudden and powerful thunderstorms occurred during the flood emergency that created flash flooding. The flash flooding would cause levees to give and break. However, thanks to the hourly fax updates from the contracted weather agency, EMS administration was able to make staffing adjustments hours ahead of time.

A major concern to the administration during the flood emergency was still the primary role of EMS: expedient response times on the streets. July and

August are traditionally the busiest time of the year for St. Louis EMS. It is not uncommon to receive over 250 calls per day, resulting in 175 transports to a hospital. Therefore, the administration could not lose focus of normal street operations. An operational "Status 5" was declared by the Chief. This was the first time that St. Louis EMS invoked a "Status 5." This meant:

1. sick leave and emergency vacation requests were denied,
2. mandatory overtime could be utilized,
3. 9-1-1 calls for minor emergencies were referred to other agencies,
4. patients were transported to the closest, most appropriate emergency receiving facility and not to the hospital of their choice,
5. hospital diversion requests were not honored, and
6. EMS personnel were subject to emergency recall on their off days.

"Status 5" proved successful. July response times averaged 6.8 minutes from the receipt of the call. In July EMS ran 6,083 9-1-1 calls and transported 3,773 patients, including flood patients. "Status 5" resulted in approximately a 20% reduction in responses and patients.

Dignitary Visits

As with any calamity, dignitary visits from elected officials and VIPs are inevitable. During the flood emergency, St. Louis received visits from such individuals as the Reverend Jesse Jackson, Bishop Desmond Tutu, numerous elected officials, and Vice President Albert Gore. It was not necessary for EMS to provide medical coverage to the dignitaries except for the Vice President in response to a request by the Secret Service. Vice President Albert Gore visited the St. Louis area in mid-July to view the devastation and efforts to control the destruction. To cover the event, a special operations tactical unit was assigned to the visit of the Vice President.

Documentation

On July 25, the city of St. Louis was declared a disaster area by President Clinton. With the declaration, federal funding would become available for reimbursement of expenses from the Federal Emergency Management Agency (FEMA). Therefore, it became necessary to maintain detailed records on all employee hours, mileage, and fuel used for all vehicles, supplies that needed to be purchased, or any other operational or administrative expense. The basic rule was to document when in doubt.

Conclusion

The flood throughout the midwest and St. Louis is described as a "once every three hundred year" flood. Over 45 people died as a result of the flooding throughout the midwest. Thankfully, no one died and no serious injuries resulted in St. Louis as a result of the flood. The lack of serious injuries or deaths can be attributed to good pre-planning, the predictability of the flood, the capability of dealing with most situations that arose—and luck. Being a paramedic in a large urban city can bring out cynicism when observing deaths from violence and crime. However, the reaffirmation in humanity was apparent when countless volunteers responded to the call for help. Those who could not sandbag donated food, money, clothes, and their time in shelters. The desire and longing to help a person in need was extraordinary.

When the "Great Flood of 1993" is over and done, critiques will show St. Louis EMS's shortcomings. But those critiques will also show that man took on nature and survived. At the time of this article, Gary Ludwig was the Deputy Chief of EMS for the city of St. Louis. He was the incident commander responsible for the entire flood operation in St. Louis. Several months after the completion of flood operations in St. Louis, he accepted a position as the Chief Paramedic for the St. Louis Fire Department. In April of 1997, St. Louis EMS was merged into the St. Louis Fire Department and Gary now serves as the EMS Bureau Chief.

Gary is also an elected EMS Executive Board member of the International Association of Fire Chiefs. He has a total of 20 years EMS and fire experience in the city of St. Louis. Gary sits on several state and national emergency service boards, editorial advisory boards of several professional trade journals, the faculty of several colleges, and the adjunct faculty of the National Fire Academy. He lectures frequently at EMS and fire conferences nationally, has a Master's Degree in Management, and is a licensed paramedic in the State of Missouri.

ON THE JOB IN COLONIAL HEIGHTS, VIRGINIA

By Dennis L. Rubin, Battalion Chief, Chesterfield Fire Department, Chesterfield, VA

On August 6, 1993, the central Virginia region was assaulted by a killer tornado. The class III tornado developed out of the west at about 1338 hours, without any warning (See Table A1-1 for categories of tornadoes.) Only after receiving damage and eyewitness reports, did area officials realize that a path of death and destruction was cut along the James and Appomattox River basins. In its wake, four people lay dead, hundreds were injured, and over 65 million dollars of property was damaged. The cities of Colonial Heights and Petersburg took direct hits, causing tremendous destruction. Two other communities, Chesterfield and Hopewell, were smacked by glancing blows. The public safety response to this disaster is probably unparalleled in the history of the Commonwealth of Virginia. Over 1,000 responders from some 60 plus agencies would be used to restore order and begin the recovery process. This article will take a detailed look at the incident management structure, strategy, and tactics that were implemented to make sense out of total chaos.

Emergency calls for assistance spiked as soon as the tornado touched down. The alarms ranged from wires down to automobile accidents to building collapses. Due to the high volume of alarm activity, emergency response resources were spread thin. Because of this resource situation, only one engine, two ambulances, and one command officer were dispatched to the Wal-Mart building collapse. The initial size-up indicated that it was a major incident. The Wal-Mart collapse turned out to be the most serious incident of many that the tornado caused. Deputy Chief Edward Snyder of Colonial Heights Fire Department assumed incident command and implemented the initial action plan (See Table A1-2 for more about the Colonial Heights Department.) The first two objectives were to assess the situation and request mutual aid assistance.

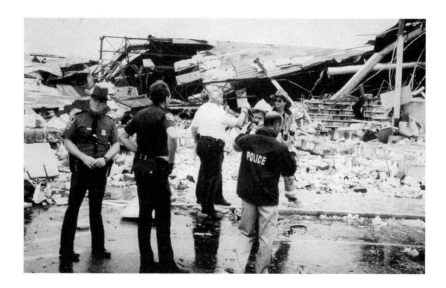

The first scenes at this collapse were hard to comprehend. About 40% of the building lay in total ruins. There were some 150 to 200 people inside the store just prior to the collapse. The building's electrical power went out and occupants indicated that sales associates and shoppers had only a few seconds' notice to brace for the impending disaster. Instantly the store occupants became victims and most needed emergency medical care. Included in this group of unlucky souls was an off-duty Chesterfield firefighter, Kenny Aliceburg. Kenny clung to one of the roof support columns for his life. The noise was deafening and the confusion tremendous, as the structure crumbled. Firefighter Aliceburg, being uninjured, helped with the evacuation and medical treatment process. Miraculously the lion's share of injuries were priority 2s and 3s. There were two priority 4 patients and less than ten priority 1 victims. One of the priority 1 patients would expire at the hospital shortly after transport.

The building was a typically large discount store. It was type II construction, noncombustible, primarily steel frame with brick veneer. The occupancy measured 385 feet (across) by 295 feet (deep) for a total of 113,000 square feet of floor space. The building was classified one story, however the ceiling height was 30 feet to allow for high-pile storage. The building consisted of 72 bays (the span from one load-bearing column to another). Twenty-seven of them were missing or destroyed after

Table A1-1 Tornado F-Scale*

CATEGORY	WINDS/SPEED	DAMAGED
CLASS I	72–112mph	Moderate damage. Roofs peeled off; windows broken; trees snapped; trailers moved or overturned.
CLASS II	113–157mph	Considerable damage. Roofs torn off; weak structures and trailers demolished; trees uprooted; cars blown off road.
CLASS III	158–206mph	Roofs and some walls torn off well-constructed houses; some rural buildings demolished; car-lifted and crumbled.
CLASS IV	207–260mph	Houses leveled leaving piles of debris; cars thrown some distance.
CLASS V	261–318mph	Well-built houses lifted clear off foundation and carried a considerable distance and disintegrated.

*Fujita Scale

Table A1-2 About the Department

Colonial Heights, Virginia. Chief A. G. Moore, Jr.

Personnel	12 career and 80 volunteer members
Apparatus	2 engine companies
Population	16,500
Area Served	8 square miles

the tornado hit. The winds ripped a wide path from the front of the store by the main entrance to the rear of the building. Further, there was another area of collapse towards side "D" of the structure that was not connected to the primary damage area. The belief is that the tornado spawned "baby" tornados, and one of these caused the separate pancake collapse.

The parking lot was a small-scaled disaster on its own. Over 100 vehicles were tossed about like so much confetti. The glass from almost all the vehicles now lay in the parking lot. Access to the building was severely limited due to the numbers of wrecked and piled-up vehicles. Early into the incident, a fleet of tow trucks was required to move the wreckage so that apparatus and heavy equipment would have access. The tornado's energy lifted forty-foot trailers and smashed them into the loading dock bays. The resemblance was more warzone like, rather than new suburban shopping mall.

As help arrived, the command structure was expanded to manage the operating resources. The unified command process would be aggressively exercised to coordinate the many jurisdictions that work together under one action plan. Due to the volume of resources from the Chesterfield Fire Department (see Table A1-3), Senior Battalion Chief Paul Shorter was appointed Deputy Incident Command. The next tactical objective was to gain scene control and support emergency medical operations. There were scores of people (sales associates, shoppers, and passers-by) who were working adamantly to remove as much debris as possible to locate trapped victims. These people reacted like an "ant pile" on a fresh piece of bread. They worked feverishly, in a disjointed and uncoordinated fashion. This freelance action was initiated in the collapse zone (of course) without any regard for personal safety. Live electrical equipment, leaking natural gas pipelines, releases of hazardous materials (pesticides), and secondary collapse were of great concern. The well-meaning citizens had to be removed and checked for injuries. Next, the building utilities had

Table A1-3 Resources Deployed

• 12 Engines	• 6 Special Units
• 4 Ladders	• 2 Haz Mat Units
• 4 Heavy Rescues	• 1 Mobile Surgical
• 700 Fire/Rescue Personnel	• 4 Track Hoes
• 29 Ambulances	• 100 Wreckers
• 4 Helicopters	• 11 Dump Trucks
• 8 Command Officers	• 5 Ten-Ton Cranes
• 250 Soldiers	• 3 Back Loaders

to be secured from street disconnects. The hazardous materials were identified by pre-plans and evaluated by the regional level III Haz Mat response team from Henrico County Fire Department. The team leader, Captain Floyd Greene, indicated that the dangerous commodities were in one of the few areas of the building that was left intact, posing no threat.

Once the scene and hazards were controlled, a primary search was organized and implemented. The building was divided into three sectors. Two companies (eight firefighters) were assigned to each rescue sector under the direction of Lt. John Crosby of the Chesterfield Fire Department. The objectives for the rescue sectors were to perform a primary search (mostly visual), identify any additional hazards, and mark locations of the facilities. This was a slow, difficult job. Upon completion, the rescue sectors located two facilities and were able to search about 70% of the building. The remaining 30% of the floor space was not accessible to the rescuers. The request for specialized resources was generated by the rescue sectors. Seven search dog teams were deployed to support the effort. The dog teams from Dogs East were able to arrive early into the situation. They conducted three or four building searches, confirming the primary "all clear."

Simultaneously the emergency medical care plan was now in full swing. Triage, treatment, and transportation sectors were established. Many of the injured left the scene after medical treatment was received and, in some cases, without even being checked by emergency medical care providers. A large number of these folks transported themselves to area hospitals. This self-transportation added to the confusion of tracking patient information. In one case, a person drove himself to one of the local emergency rooms. Upon his arrival, he realized that his automobile had been significantly damaged, causing the doors to be jammed. The hospital emergency room personnel had to call for the Fire Department to respond to the parking lot and extricate the gentleman. Because of the rapid treatment and movement of patients (planned and unplanned), triage tags could not be effectively used.

Fortunately many ambulances and other emergency medical resources were readily available. Due to the level of response and minimal number of seriously injured patients, the bulk of the emergency medical care was over within the first hour. Some 185 people were transported to only two local hospitals. The disproportionate distribution of patients from this incident was of some concern to local hospital officials. However, after investigation, it was learned that a significant number of the injured drove themselves to the hospitals. Also, the major highway (Interstate 95) was backed up for miles. This traffic jam eliminated all hospitals north of the incident as transport alternatives. The ability to treat, package, and transport this volume of customers within sixty minutes stands as a tremendous tribute to the regional effort and response to this disaster. The emergency medical care providers distinguished themselves as outstanding that day.

With the primary search and patient care complete, the incident action plan was updated. The focus now shifted to long-term operations, including removal of the two fatalities, searching the remaining 30% of the building with shoring techniques, removing valuables (weapons, drugs, money, and computer records), and scene security. While the Federal Emergency Management Agency's Urban Search and Rescue Task Force was in transit, manual debris removal got underway. Heavy equipment that was called for about one hour into the incident was now pressed into service.

The heavy equipment would remove the large slabs of falling building components. Once lifted outside the collapse zone, the materials were loaded into a fleet of waiting dump trucks for removal. Once the large items were taken away, hand crews would clear the topical debris, ensuring that no victims remained. This was difficult and primitive work. There was a high degree of danger working in this environment. The heavy equipment was noisy and vibrated significantly. Because of these factors, the remaining walls and roof assemblies had to be constantly evaluated for movement. The movement would be a sign of impending secondary collapse.

In order to perform the tremendous amount of detailed work, the military was called. Soldiers from the Fort Lee Army Post, under the command of the Lieutenant General Samuel Wakefield, were activated early and remained throughout the incident. To maintain communications, crew integrity, and personal safety, the soldiers were divided into crews of five and assigned to a qualified firefighter. Further, the military set up a "tent city" to support their operation. They were completely self-contained from food to sanitary facilities to sleeping quarters. As midnight approached, the FEMA Urban Search and Rescue Task Force arrived. Interestingly, this call made several "firsts" with the Virginia Beach USAR team. It was their "maiden voyage" as well as the first ground activation, the first in-state response, and the first time a federal USAR team was requested by the state government. The USAR team began to provide initial technical support. The task force leader, District Chief Melvin Mathias of Virginia Beach Fire Department, concurred with our incident action plan. The USAR team started their operation by shoring the collapsed area. Once shored, these areas were searched for victims. To ensure accuracy, the search dogs were sent into the now accessed areas. Fortunately there were no additional victims remaining in the building.

It took about eighteen hours to completely search the building. With the life safety priority met, emphasis was placed on debris removal, with great concern for the potential Haz Mat, release. The Wal-Mart organization took an active role in the decision-making process at this point. In fact, throughout the operation the Wal-Mart management team was extremely helpful.

In summary, there were several major operational highlights that I would like to mention

- No Firefighter Injuries
- The Organization and Unification of the Command Structure
- The EMS Operations
- The Search/Extrication Operations
- The Logistical Support
- The Federal Emergency Management Agency USAR Task Force
- The Disaster Plan Implementation and EOC Operations

Finally, I would like to point out the lessons that were learned or reinforced at this incident:

1. **Staging**—The initial staging area was established too close to the incident, with many people attempting to self-deploy and "visit" the Operations section area. Once the staging function was moved and better organized, the dangerous practice of self-deployment was resolved. The need for a separate staging area was never more present.

2. **ICS Training**—Some of the agencies that attended the incident were unfamiliar with the incident command system process. The lack of knowledge negatively impacted the effectiveness of the resources on location. On many occasions, "on the spot" ICS training was conducted to be able to deploy resources.

3. **Urban Search and Rescue**—The Federal Emergency Management Agency's Urban Search and Rescue Task Force provided invaluable help. They were able to safely and efficiently conduct a primary search of the building that was not accessible to us. However, two areas presented themselves that could have been improved. When the USAR team arrived, there was a delay in their deployment. The reason for this delay was the request for assistance from the Old Towne Petersburg incident. The best way to have resolved this conflict would have been to request the USAR team from Fairfax County, as well. One team should have been dispatched to each jurisdiction. The other area for improvement is understanding the USAR team's capability, resources, and needs. Not much, if any, information has been provided about how the team operates.

4. **Control Air Space**—Due to this newsworthy incident, a great number of media agencies covered the story. As part of the media operations, a large volume of aircraft was dispatched to the Wal-Mart scene. At various points, as many as ten aircraft were spotted in close proximity. The number of air operations around the incident increased the risk to the ground forces. As well, they added to the confusion and noise problems.

5. **Media Relations**—The appointment of a Public Information Officer was somewhat late in the process. With local and national media arriving quickly at this incident, we should have placed more emphasis on a media release strategy. Regular media briefings should have been held throughout the incident. The lack of early press releases frustrated the media. Several media representatives contacted me at the Operations area for information. I expressed the need for them to stand behind the barrier line and PIO would contact them. The media perceive that they have a "right to know" and therefore nearly demand information. This stress factor could have been relieved and we could have utilized the media coverage to our advantage. Once established and supported, the media plan went very smoothly. At one point, the media were taken on guided tours of the destruction area.

This was a highly publicized and scrutinized event. Local, state, and national elected officials attended and reviewed our operation in detail. Only through the implementation and utilization of the incident command system could this massive amount of resources have been managed properly. The responders worked incredibly hard and ICS was successful.

Some of the Agencies Operating at This Incident

Colonial Heights Fire Department
Chesterfield Fire Department
Chesterfield County EMS
Richmond Fire Department
Henrico Fire Department
Henrico County EMS
Prince County Fire Department
Dinwiddie County Fire Department
U. S. Army—Ft. Lee
A & B Ambulance Service
Hanover Volunteer EMS
Virginia Beach Fire Department

HIGH-RISE FIRE IN WILMINGTON, DELAWARE

By Deputy Chief Lawrence Tan, New Castle County EMS Division, Department of Public Safety, New Castle, DE

System Overview

The New Castle County EMS Division is a county, municipal-based agency. The agency is responsible for the delivery of out-of-hospital care to the 437 square miles of the county, including the incorporated and unincorporated areas, serving a population of approximately 468,000.

New Castle County EMS Division has an authorized staff of 97 personnel, which includes 5 EMS supervisors, 72 paramedics, and 14 emergency medical technicians. The executive staff includes a chief and 2 deputy chiefs of EMS. The division usually fields 7 paramedic units and one BLS ambulance on a 24-hour basis, and two additional BLS ambulances on a scheduled, Monday through Friday basis.

Emergency medical services are currently provided in a tiered response configuration with the county volunteer fire service, which provides basic life support ambulance capabilities. American Medical Response provides a contracted, basic life support service to the city of Wilmington, in conjunction with the New Castle County EMS paramedic services.

The city of Wilmington has a career fire department consisting of approximately 130 personnel that staff 6 engine companies, 2 ladder companies, and a heavy rescue squad.

Incident Overview

On Thursday, April 2, 1997, the county emergency communications center received a report of a building fire in the Delaware Trust Building at 902 North

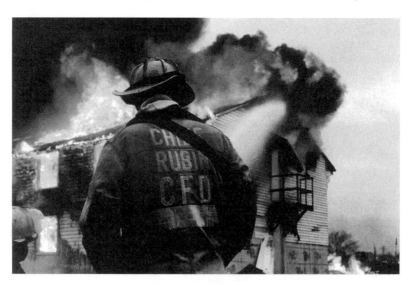

Market Street. The caller, a security guard for the facility, reported smoke on the 14th floor. The initial Wilmington Fire Department apparatus reported smoke conditions on the upper floors. New Castle County Medic 1 responded to the incident after the initial reports of a possible "working" alarm, and established an EMS staging area at 10th and Market Streets.

Wilmington Fire Department crews continued to report heavy smoke and heat conditions on multiple floors of the 22-floor building, prompting the deputy chief of operations to declare a "general alarm" for the incident at approximately 2139 hours. The general alarm recalls all off-duty Wilmington Fire Department personnel, places all reserve apparatus in service, and brings in the volunteer fire service from the county to cover the vacant city fire stations.

At 2151 hours the incident commander requested an EMS assignment of 2 paramedic units, 4 basic life support ambulances, and an EMS supervisor for medical support. The on-duty EMS shift commander and EMS staff duty officer, a deputy chief of EMS, were notified to respond to the scene. All EMS units responded to the designated staging area at 10th and Market Streets. An exterior EMS triage/treatment area was established in a pedestrian walkway in the front of the structure. The triage area was placed in a manner that would not impede access or egress to the building by firefighters, but was in direct proximity to the main entry and exit point to the building. A perimeter was established by the Wilmington Police Department, essentially closing the pedestrian walkway for the duration of the incident. The EMS shift commander was originally assigned as the staging officer, but was later relocated and assigned as the interior EMS triage/rehab sector officer.

On arrival, the EMS deputy chief assumed responsibility for EMS group operations, while the EMS shift commander obtained a detailed accounting of all EMS personnel assigned to the incident. The deputy chief proceeded to the incident command post at 9th and Market Streets and obtained a briefing from the incident commander. The IC advised that units operating on the interior were reporting heavy fire and smoke conditions on the 13th through 16th floors, with smoke conditions on the 17th through 22nd floors. Further, he advised that the interior firefighting personnel were reporting no progress on the interior operations.

The IC requested that EMS personnel be assigned to the 12th floor staging area of the operation as a "forward" triage and rehab area. One paramedic crew (2 paramedics) and two BLS crews (2 EMTs each) were assigned to the interior triage. Paramedics used bottled spring water in the building to rehydrate firefighters, and provided medical support to firefighting units taken off line for a break. Progress reports to the EMS group commander were established at 30–45 minute intervals. Initially the paramedics reported that they were providing rehab for approximately 30 firefighters.

A short time later, the paramedics in the interior of the building reported a "light haze" of smoke on the 12th floor. The IC was immediately notified, and interior EMS operations were relocated to the 10th floor, along with the interior firefighter staging area. Additionally, a patient evacuation and EMS supply route was established using the only functional elevator in the building. The patient evacuation plan enabled EMS group personnel to effect a timely removal of any firefighters who needed to be transported to a medical facility, and provided a coordinated transfer of care to exterior EMS personnel.

The Wilmington Fire Department had committed all of its resources to this operation, and had requested the following additional apparatus from the county volunteer fire service: 8 engines, with an additional 5 engines for cover-up in vacant Wilmington stations, 2 additional ladder companies, 6 additional rescues for air support, and 3 additional BLS ambulances. Later 4 of the cover-up engines would be assigned to the incident, resulting in 4 additional engines being requested from the county volunteer fire service for station coverage (17 total engines brought to the city of Wilmington).

On April 5, 1997, the Delaware Emergency Management Agency issued an "advisory" regarding the potential for asbestos and polychlorinated biphenyls (PCBs) at this incident. Subsequent testing for PCBs proved negative; however, asbestos was found to be present. The detailed accounting of all EMS units and personnel assigned to the incident permitted the EMS Division to document the potential exposure to asbestos and take the necessary post-exposure action. The EMS Division also forwarded copies of all available information to any outside agencies that participated in EMS group operations at this incident.

Results

The EMS Division was providing medical support to an estimated 250 firefighters during an extended firefighting operation that lasted approximately 8 hours. The medical support operation included continuous hydration of the firefighting force, and other routine care such as eye irrigation. The EMS group treated seven firefighters and transported five to area hospitals, including a firefighter with chest pain who was admitted to the intensive care unit.

Additional EMS Division personnel and another EMS shift commander were activated to handle the continued demand for 9-1-1 system EMS requests.

Some Lessons Learned

The designation of an EMS staging area by the first arriving paramedics unit was of great assistance in coordinating the response of additional EMS units to the incident, and enabled us to maintain continuous accountability and tracking of EMS personnel assigned to the incident. This information proved to be valuable when the issue of potential exposure to hazardous materials was presented several days after the incident. The use of a "joint command post" facilitated the transmission of information to the EMS group and enabled us to provide immediate notification of any firefighting personnel who were being transported from the scene.

The designation of a single EMS group commander permitted the coordination of supply and/or personnel requests. Additional supplies, such as oxygen administration equipment, towels, blankets, etc., could be requested and coordinated with area hospitals. In fact, two local hospitals provided after-hour access to their laundry facilities in order to provide additional towels and blankets to the scene. The EMS group commander was also able to verify that the requesting persons had received the items. It would have been helpful for an aide to be assigned to the EMS group commander at the incident command post. The aide would have been helpful in tracking the status of EMS units and personnel, monitoring communications, and maintaining documentation of the incident for the post-incident/after action report.

EMS units and personnel should have a designated point of contact when arriving on scene, and be issued specific instructions on their responsibility during the operation. This is particularly true during multiple-agency operations, where unit and personnel accountability are a potential problem.

The use of the incident command system for EMS operations at the incident facilitated communications and provided a more effective management structure for EMS group operations at this incident. The ICS also identified the lines of communication for the duration of the incident. It is imperative that documentation of EMS group activities take place either at the communications center and/or at the incident scene. This documentation can prove to be vital in the event of worker's compensation investigations or subsequent post-incident analysis of agency activities. In our situation, the EMS progress reports documented unit and personnel activity throughout the operation. Additionally we were able to identify exactly when firefighters presented themselves to EMS personnel for care and the time they were subsequently transported to a hospital.

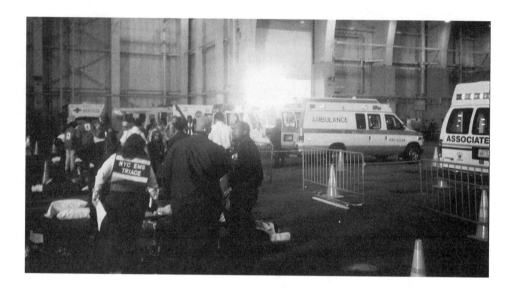

INCIDENT IN WESTWOOD, CALIFORNIA

By James P. Denney

In the evening, the day before the 1984 Olympics opened, Westwood, California was crowded with celebrants anticipating the Olympic opening. The small village borders the UCLA campus and consists of shops, restaurants, coffeehouses, and ice cream parlors. On warm nights like this one, it is not unusual for a thousand or more students and residents to stroll the sidewalk, meet at small cafes, or simply socialize while enjoying a walk through town.

On this particular evening a young man, under the influence of PCP, decided to drive his car at high speed down a sidewalk crowded with an estimated 700+ men, women, and children, including Olympic athletes.

Needless to say, we were presented with an immediate event of magnitude having several components. Not only were we faced with a multi-casualty incident of unknown proportions, a crime scene and a multi-cultural polyglot tourist population, but the international press would be present to observe our actions and to comment on how effective our system would be in mitigating this catastrophe.

The first calls received by the PSAP indicated that a motorist had crashed into a bus kiosk at the southern end of the block, injuring approximately eight people. This call resulted in the dispatch of two rescue ambulances, a fire task force (truck company and two-piece engine company with a total of ten personnel), a Battalion Chief (BC), EMS District Commander, and a police unit for traffic control.

Upon arrival the scene was bedlam. The task force and EMS personnel immediately began assessing the extent of the incident and the triage of victims. The

Battalion Chief established a command post and implemented the multi-casualty incident plan. The EMS District Commander arrived within a few minutes, was briefed by the BC, and began the establishment of a Medical Division.

Three additional rescue ambulances and another task force established immediate, delayed, and minor care holding areas, and an ambulance control officer was assigned along with a patient transportation recorder. A separate radio frequency in addition to the med-net was allocated to the Medical Division.

As additional victims made themselves known and the incident began to expand, additional resources and personnel were requested. I arrived about 25 minutes into the incident and was immediately given the responsibility for incident site survey. (My initial assignment was to "360" the incident to ensure we had accurate information on the size and scope of the problem.)

By the time I had completed my survey, I had determined that the incident was linear and extended approximately 550 feet to the north in an eight-foot-wide corridor. I estimated that there were an additional 60 to 80 victims in various categories, extending the length of the incident. By now, the site was in pandemonium with convergent volunteers and spectators hampering rescue efforts and medical operations. I reported my findings to the Incident Commander, and additional resources were requested and dispatched to a staging area to the east of the incident. An ambulance staging area was established in the center of the incident, where a side street gave access and a traffic flow pattern was developed. A police command post was established adjacent to the Incident Commander and appropriate crowd control measures were taken.

The hospital system for the area was contacted by the local Medical Alert Center, and bed availability was obtained in addition to "blanket treatment orders." A medical cache was ordered and delivered to the Medical Division, where it was used to care for patients and to restock ambulances. (A medical cache provided BLS level supplies and equipment to treat 50 casualties.) An equipment recovery center was established adjacent to the Medical Division, where recovered backboards, traction splints, and other equipment were stored by returning ambulances.

Once the scope of the incident was determined and adequate resources were on scene, all patients requiring attention were processed (treated, packaged, and transported) within 48 minutes. The entire incident took less than two hours to complete. The Incident Command System provided a sequential, ordered, management tool that guaranteed a disciplined response to an otherwise chaotic event.

THE AMTRAK SUNSET LIMITED DISASTER IN MOBILE, ALABAMA

By Paul R. Smith, Fire Service Captain, REMTP, Mobile Fire-Rescue Department, Mobile, AL

September 22, 1993, a day that will never be forgotten by the members of the Mobile Fire-Rescue Department or the community as a whole. This was the day Mobile was indoctrinated into the world of Mass Casualty Disasters.

The AmTrak Sunset Limited, a coast-to-coast passenger train traveling from California to Florida, was carrying 206 passengers and crew members as she made her way south. While passing through New Orleans, LA, she was delayed for 33 minutes for AC and toilet repairs. There are many who say these 33 minutes doomed her. She arrived in Mobile, AL 30 minutes behind schedule. As she cleared the CSX railyard heading north out of Mobile, she gained speed to approximately 72 MPH, on her way to meet with destiny.

Meanwhile the tugboat MV Mauvilla was also moving north on the Mobile River. It was one of those foggy Mobile mornings along the river. The MV Mauvilla was piloted by Willie Odom, as testimony has shown, slowly making the trip north on the river.

Just north of Mobile in the middle of the river sits an island, Twelve Mile Island. At the north end of the island, the river forks. To the right you have the continuation of the Mobile River. To the left is big Bayou Canot, a navigable waterway, not for commercial use. For approximately one-half mile into the bayou, there is a railroad bridge, which, at that time, was not marked by lights and sits approximate-

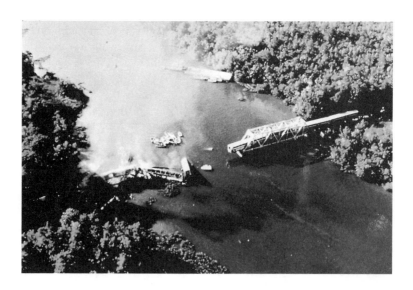

ly six feet off the water. The MV Mauvilla made the wrong turn! As the Mauvilla moved deeper into Bayou Canot, testimony has shown, Mr. Odom notes that the heal of his tow disappeared and he felt a bump. The rest of the story is a true tragedy.

The first call for help was received by an E-911 call taker at 0301 hours. Mr. Warren Carr from CSX railroad called and advised, "We have a passenger train derailed at the Bayou Sara drawbridge. People are in the water and cars are on fire." As you can imagine, the next 18 minutes in the E-911 communications center were very confusing. The operators were unfamiliar with the locations on the river and in the delta. They are used to taking street addresses or names. In a desperate attempt to locate the reported accident and to confirm its existence, the operators called all of the surrounding jurisdictions: Prichard, Chickasaw, Saraland and the most northern jurisdiction to Mobile, Satsuma. To make matters even worse, the call-back number Mr. Carr gave was hooked up to a recording. This made the stress level in the E-911 center even greater for the operators. Now unable to even confirm the accident, the operators continued their frantic search for information on the accident. The company officer on duty at Fire Station 21 was called for information on the area. All he could assist with was advising the operators that they respond in the area when needed. After several more calls to the surrounding jurisdictions, the location was narrowed down to the Mobile River, then the northeast corner of the city limits.

The operator called the fire boat captain to ask if he had responded to Twelve Mile Island. At 0320 the initial dispatch was sent: "Attention Engine 21, Engine 14, Engine 1, Truck 4, District 1 Chief, and Fire Boat 2, for a possible train derailment at Bayou Sara drawbridge at the Mobile River." Eighteen minutes had elapsed from the receipt of the initial call.

I was the EMS Shift Commander that tragic morning. I responded prior to being dispatched along with Fire Rescue 14. While en route to the incident, Fire Boat 2 confirmed the accident via the marine radio. A Scott Paper Company (now Kimberly Clark) tug from the Scott fleet was on scene along with the MV Mauvilla. District 1 Chief Vernon Hall advised all units to stage at the Saraland Fire Department on HWY 43.

While I was en route, fire alarm called me and advised that we had 226 people on board the train. With this information I started notifying other agencies from which I felt we would need assistance. I first notified the University of South Alabama Medical Center, our regional level one trauma center, and the South Flite of the incident, to place the helicopter on standby to notify all area hospitals in Mobile and Baldwin Counties. Second, I notified Newmans Ambulance Service. Off-duty Firemedic Ed Wood was the supervisor on duty. I told him to start two ALS units, including himself, to Saraland, notify all private ambulance companies in the area, and to call in off-duty personnel. Next I contacted Dr. Ballard for Medical Control at Springhill Memorial Hospital, which the Mobile Fire-Rescue Department uses as our Medical Control Hospital. As the units started arriving in the staging area in Saraland, Chief Hall advised we would be unable to reach the scene through Saraland. He had been led approximately 1.5 miles into the area by a Saraland police officer, hoping to locate a land entrance to the incident scene. All units were ordered to relocate to the Cochran Bridge at Scott Paper Company on Bay Bridge Road, which sits on the Mobile River. En route to Scott, I called a fire alarm to notify the EMS chief and to call CSX to put together a rescue train, flat beds or box cars, and an engine—anything that could transport crews and equipment up and patients back.

Fire boat 2 arrived at the derailment scene at approximately 0400 hours, over one hour into the incident. South Flite advised just prior to the arrival of the fire boat: "They could see cars in the water, a large fire, and possible survivors in the water and on the tracks."

The command post was established by me at Scott Paper at 0410 hours. The Incident Command System was established, all Chief Officers were to be notified by fire alarm, EMA was notified, and all off-duty Firemedics were to be called into the staging area. Initially we used four sectors of the ICS: Operations, which included Task Force 1, two engine companies, one ladder company, and two fire rescues (for a total of twelve firefighters, three Firemedics, and one intermediate EMT); Planning; Logistics; and Medical. Finance was added later as staff personnel arrived in staging.

Task Force 1 loaded the rescue train to start towards the derailment. WKRG TV slipped a cameraman on board the train. He produced the only early photos and documentation of the scene and events. Ambulance staging, landing zones, and fire apparatus staging officers were appointed as additional resources arrived. When I was relieved of command by EMS Chief Byrd and then Deputy Chief Dean, I moved into my normal role as EMS Sector Officer. In this sector I had responsibility for extrication, triage, treatment, transport in, and rehab, both on site and, the remote areas. As additional personnel arrived at the staging area, I was able to assign people to start setting up the main triage area, rehab, and a possible, temporary morgue.

When the rescue train arrived on scene, "The people were waiting on the tracks," Fire Service Driver REMTP George Watson advised later in a debriefing session. "When the light came on, they got up and started walking towards us in silence," he said.

The fire boat activities included initial search and rescue, but all victims were removed from the water either by the tugs or by assistance from each other. No search of the cars was completed initially due to the lack of manpower on the fireboat which had responded with the usual three-man crew. The scene was described by Captain Greg Foster from the fire boat as "Something you would only see in a movie!" The fire consisted of three parts: (1) the train contents, three engines, the baggage car, and the crew coach; (2) a large area fuel fire caused by the ruptured fuel cell carrying 2500 to 3000 gallons of diesel fuel; and (3) the creosote bridge pilings and cross ties. All fires were allowed to burn, with only minimal suppression activities. This was because the fire was providing the only light in the bayou, except for three spot lights on the tugs and fire boat.

At day break, the reality of the incident set in. It was learned that we had one car half submerged, one car completely submerged, and dozens missing. The fire that was allowed to burn stubbornly persisted. The fire boat was unable to move around for fear of hitting a missing victim.

I was advised that the rescue train was departing the scene at 0530 hours, with 126 patients on board. It arrived at the main triage area, where the patients were retriaged, their names recorded, and then they were transported by ambulance or bus to local hospitals. I had made the decision that anyone off the train would be transported to the hospital for observation, regardless of a complaint of injury or not. I decided this because everyone who went into the water was contaminated with diesel fuel and I felt, emotionally they all needed to talk to someone.

A kink was thrown into my smooth-running EMS Sector when Task Force 1 advised that we had 28 victims coming in by tug to the east side of the river at Scott Fleet's Dock at 0615 hours. A second triage area was then established and these patients were triaged and transported accordingly. At this same time, I was advised by fire alarm of five patients at the United States Coast Guard Aviation Training Center Base at Bates Field, approximately 20 miles west of our location. They had been airlifted from the scene and flown there. These patients were removed from the north side of the accident. Four ambulances responding from the south part of the county were diverted to Bates and these patients were transported.

At 0640 hours the rescue train was loaded once again with personnel and extrication equipment for a second trip to the scene. Dr. John McMahon, our Fire Physician and Medical Control Physician, along with two additional physicians from the University of South Alabama Medical Center, went on the second trip. By approximately 0720 hours, Task Force 1 advised that we had no remaining treatable patients and that we needed eighty to one hundred body bags.

MFRD's activities continued on scene and at the command post. By 0730 hours, overhaul operations commenced. Divers from Lee Diving Company started searching the submerged cars. MFRD and Mobile Police Department photographers and Identification Sector arrived on the scene. At approximately 0750 hours the last patient was transported to the hospital from triage. That was the same time that the first patient was being discharged from the hospital.

When the first body was recovered, the need for a temporary morgue became apparent. A barge was used for an on-site, temporary morgue. The barge was used as an ID section and Alabama Department of Forensic Sciences could set up at the Port of Chickasaw. By 1130 hours national and international news media were at the Port of Chickasaw.

MFRD's three primary activities were: (1) to continue fire overhaul; (2) to retrieve and remove victims; and (3) to man the temporary morgue barge. Within the first 24 hours, most of the passengers and crew had been accounted for. The duration of body recovery lasted three days.

The three engineers in the lead engine were recovered on Friday, 48 hours after the accident, buried fifty-seven feet down in the north river bank. The final count of victims was 206. 159 patients were triaged, treated, and transported to local hospitals. Forty-two passengers and 5 crew members lost their lives that foggy Mobile morning. This became the worst AmTrak accident in U.S. history and the largest mass casualty disaster ever to occur in Mobile. Every agency involved should be commended on its performance.

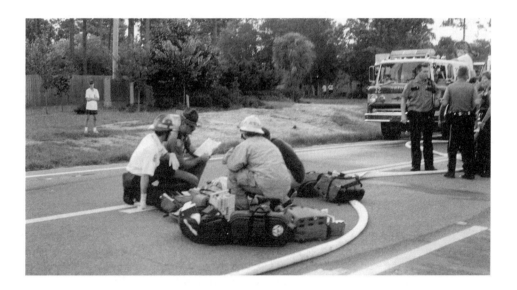

I-10 BAYWAY ACCIDENT IN MOBILE, ALABAMA

By Paul R. Smith, Fire Service Captain, REMTP, Mobile Fire-Rescue Department, Mobile, AL

Monday, March 20, 1996, 0620 hours. My partner, Firemedic G.A. Tony Rutland, and I rolled out of bed, 40 minutes until shift change at Central Fire Station, Fire Rescue 3. The night went by with only one minor glitch, a run around 2100 hours. As we slept this morning, the fog rolled in over the bay and causeway, spilling slightly into downtown Mobile. Now as we prepared to be relieved of duty, the morning routine would soon be broken by yet another run.

At 0637 hours the alarm sounded for Fire Rescue 3 and Engine 2. There was a wreck with injuries on I-10 eastbound between the tunnel and the causeway. When I made it to the truck, Tony had checked en route already. I looked at Tony and told him, "This is probably going to be another minor accident which causes us to get off late." Oh, how wrong I was to be about that. Late yes, minor no. We respond to many calls on the Bayway, many of which I would say are minor. Yes, some are very bad accidents, but not at this time of the morning. The I-10 Bayway spans seven miles over the Mobile Bay and river delta connecting Mobile and Baldwin Counties.

En route we noticed some mild fog conditions in the downtown area, and as we entered the I-10 George Wallace Tunnel, I remember not thinking much about this at all. The area has fog on a regular basis. Going through the tunnel the procession of emergency vehicles was: Engine 2, Fire Rescue 3, and a single Mobile police car. We passed approximately 40 vehicles, including several tractor trailers, in the tunnel. Just as we exited the tunnel, Fire Rescue 3 signaled to Engine 2 that we were going to pass. As we passed, the MPD unit passed us all. This turned out to be one of the best things that could have happened.

Once out of the tunnel, there was some light fog. Again we did not pay it much attention because fog isn't out of the ordinary. Approximately a half mile east of the tunnel, the fog thickened. Visibility was approximately 50 to 60 feet, which happens on occasion. At one mile east of the tunnel visibility dropped from 50 to 60 feet to zero. The MPD unit was 12 feet in front of Fire Rescue 3, and Engine 2 was 30 feet behind us. Immediately Tony started slowing down fast. We had lost sight of the MPD unit and Engine 2. Within ten seconds we were on top of the MPD unit and the accident. Fire Rescue 3 stopped three feet from the rear bumper of the MPD unit, and Engine 2 stopped 20 feet from us.

Tony and I exited the unit at the same time Acting Captain Sam Downing and Firefighter Scott Johnson exited Engine 2. Visibility was near zero, but I could make out one jackknifed tractor trailer with three cars under it and approximately fifteen other vehicles piled into each other. Tony and I were standing approximately 10 to 15 feet in front of Engine 2, coming up with a quick game plan when a full-size pick-up truck slammed into the rear of Engine 2. As I reached for my speaker mike on my right shoulder, we heard a sound that we will never forget—the sound of air brakes locking up on a large truck. Suddenly, like out of a horror movie, we saw the tractor trailer come out of the heavy fog over behind Engine 2. Needless to say, everyone started running. The excitement level was off the scale and we were running for our lives. Tony dove over the hood of the rescue truck, I dove over the first car I came to as Firefighter Johnson did the same. For those of you who have seen the movie *The Fugitive,* you can almost see what we did. Acting Captain Downing was just able to dive back into the cab of Engine 2 as it was hit, and Jay Atchison, the driver, was holding on for the ride of his life.

Once Engine 2, which was pushed down the interstate 20 feet by the tractor trailer which was traveling at 67 MPH, stopped and we came out of hiding, I started calling for assistance. As I made sure we were all OK, I continued calling for additional assistance. On the scene initially we had two Firemedics and three firefighter EMTDs. I established command within the first minute of the incident. The decision was made to work east on the Bayway ONLY since we could hear vehicles hitting each other behind us, or west of us. Triage was initiated by myself and Firefighter Johnson. I assigned Tony to treatment. Acting Captain Downing was assigned to extricate everyone he could, as Firefighter Driver Atchison pulled a 1 3/4 inch pre-connect line off the truck for a safety line.

Within the first five minutes of the incident, I had called for four additional ALS Fire Rescue trucks, three private BLS ambulances, two engine companies, extrication, and two wreckers. I was only off by 30 to 40 wreckers from what would finally be used. At this point, I was unaware of any additional patients or exactly how large the accident was. I could only see up to the jackknifed tractor trailer, approximately 50 feet.

At the ten-minute mark of on-scene activities, we had completely used all of the immobilization equipment and most of the bandaging supplies on Fire Rescue 2. Initially I thought the accident included only 20 vehicles. It was not until I climbed on top of the jackknifed tractor trailer's cab and several people ran to me saying that people were hurt and trapped further up that I determined this was a very large-scale accident. After it was all over, it was determined that the accident covered one and a half miles of the seven-mile bridge. There was one mile of accident east, or in front of us, and a half mile of accident west, or behind us. The 40 vehicles and tractor trailers we passed in the tunnel now made up the half mile of accident behind, or west of us. This totally isolated us from additional responding units and made it impossible to transport our injured.

I decided the only way to try to get a grasp of the incident was to find the east end of the accident. I started walking and climbing over and under vehicles, heading east. District Chief John Hicks, our Training Chief, was approximately a fourth of a mile behind our location when he called Fire Alarm to completely shut down the Bayway. He then became cut off from additional units as vehicles piled in behind him. Within the first 100 to 200 feet away from Fire Rescue 3, I had discovered six patients trapped in vehicles and several injuries. I made several stops along the way, treating and assisting patients, which allowed Chief Hicks to catch up with me.

I was relieved of command by District One Chief Mike Burnson, who responded to the tunnel control room and set up a command post. This placed me in an EMS triage officer position. Chief Hicks, after 45 minutes, found the east end of the accident. By this time several units had arrived at either end and were making their way towards the middle.

By 0717 hours the MFRD had committed 26 different units to the Bayway Incident. The triage and treatment areas were manned by 12 MFRD EMTDs and Firemedics, with approximately 200 other MFRD personnel assigned to extrication, transport, rehab, search and rescue, overhaul, public information, and command staff. There were approximately 10 private BLS and ALS Mobile County and Baldwin County ambulances used, along with two Mobile Metro Buses.

A second accident occurred at approximately 0700 hours in the west-bound lanes of the Bayway. This accident was not as large as the eastbound accident the MFRD was working, but was a deadly accident. The Spanish Fort VRD in Baldwin County worked the accident which had 31 vehicles involved. There were 11 victims treated and transported to Thomas Hospital in Fairhope, Alabama. Sadly the only fatality occurred here. A woman was trapped in her car as uninjured victims attempted to remove her. The fire that she died in did not start at the time of the impact. A spark from somewhere ignited the fuel spilled on the Bayway, which claimed her life.

In all there were 193 vehicles involved in the eastbound I-10 Bayway accident and 64 confirmed patients. Twenty-nine of the patients were treated by the first arriving crews on Fire Rescue 3 and Engine 2. By 0900 hours command started releasing personnel from the incident. By 1400 hours some traffic was moving on the Bayway once again. By 1700 hours the Bayway was completely open and rush hour commuters sped, like nothing had happened just 12 hours earlier.

Lessons Learned in the AmTrak and the I-10 Bayway Incidents

1. The value of multi-agency mass casualty drills.
2. The Incident Command System or Incident Management System works.
   a. The need for a Unified Command at all large incidents with large numbers of players from different agencies.
3. The value of the Emergency Management Agency (The Human Yellow Pages).
4. Communications:

    a. Portable radios—Our VHF system was poor.
      1. Since the AmTrak incident the MFRD has gone to the 800 mhz.
      2. This did help us with the Bayway; much better communications.
    b. Cellular phone—great
      1. Bag phones
        a. They had about two hours on a battery.
        b. 12-volt outlets needed for charging and/or to use direct current.
      2. Pocket compacts
        a. Battery life short.
        b. No option for plug in after battery is dead.
      3. Have extra batteries for both radios and phones.

5. Relieve personnel frequently.
    a. Assign them different duties.
    b. Limit total time at the incident if possible.
    (No such thing as Superman or Wonder Woman).

6. Rehab.
    a. Location
    b. Food, drink and rest
    c. Restroom facilities
    (Mother Nature doesn't stop calling at a disaster.)

7. Transport officer to get supplies moving to the scene.
    a. Acquire a mode of transportation for supplies if you are not in direct contact with the command post area.
      1. At the AmTrak we were 10 miles apart in the middle of a river delta.

8. Critical Incident Stress Debriefing (CISD) is needed for everyone involved.

9. Try not to overtax your initial personnel.
    a. I tried to be command and triage at the Bayway. You can't do two jobs at one time.
    b. I only had one treatment medic and he was definitely overloaded.
    c. But remember, we are trained to do what we have to do to get the job done.

10. Never let your guard down!!!!!!!!
    a. I'm guilty of it, as is everyone.
      1. I didn't think anything would hit us on the Bayway.
      2. The people in the westbound lane accident didn't think the vehicle would become a fireball.
      3. We are all taught to check for a secure scene, which can change in a flash. Always be prepared and ready for the unexpected.

11. Remember your safety.
    a. Wear your proper personal protective gear.
    b. If you become injured, you're not helping anyone and now you're part of the problem.

12. Pace yourself.
    a. If it is a large incident and you're alone or part of a small group, work at an easy pace. If you wear yourself out, again you are now part of the problem and can't help anyone.

13. Last, a personal favorite of mine NOW!
    a. Always place the largest or heaviest rescue vehicle between you and the accident or between you and any possible threat to you.

Remember, we are out there to help protect lives and that starts with your life and those of your own personnel!!

APPENDIX II
INCIDENT MANAGEMENT FORMS

Checklist: EMS Branch Supplies
EMS IMS Chart
Checklist: Transport
Patient Disposition Data
Checklist: Triage
Checklist: Treatment
Checklist: Staging
Communications Chart
Incident Objectives

All incident management forms that have an NFES number can be ordered from the NWCC, National Fire Equipment System Catalog Part 2: Publications (NFES# 3362) National Interagency Fire Center, Great Basin Cache Supply Office, 3833 S. Development Avenue, Boise, Idaho 83705.

  Other forms can be expanded and duplicated for use in the EMS Incident Management System command cache. Forms should be inserted between sheets of one-eighth inch Plexiglass to ensure a "streetproof" checklist/command board for each IMS position. The sheets can be anchored with aluminum screwposts (office supplies). We recommend a Sanford Sharpe weatherproof marker.

EMS Branch Checklist

CHECKLIST:

EMS BRANCH

RADIO CALL SIGN: "EMS BRANCH"

SUPPLIES

1. CMD BOX
2. RADIO – PAGER
3. CELL PHONE
4. VEST
5. MARKING PENS
6. LIGHTING
7. EMS IMS CHART

Check	Item
	ENSURE SAFETY
	COORDINATE WITH INCIDENT MANAGER (COMMANDER)
	TRIAGE OFFICER
	TREATMENT OFFICER
	TRANSPORT OFFICER
	ESTABLISH TACTICAL COMMUNICATIONS CHANNELS
	MED SUPPLIES — DISASTER CACHES
	RECON ALL POSSIBLE PATIENT AREAS
	PATIENT COUNT
	ADDITIONAL AMBULANCES/RESOURCES
	(IF REQUIRED) MUTUAL AID
	DIVISIONS IF MULTIPLE PATIENT AREAS
	COORDINATE WITH OTHER BRANCH
	CALL FOR ADDITIONAL EMS MANAGERS (OFFICERS)
	RECALL OFF-DUTY PERSONNEL
	MEDEVAC (GPS COORDINATOR)

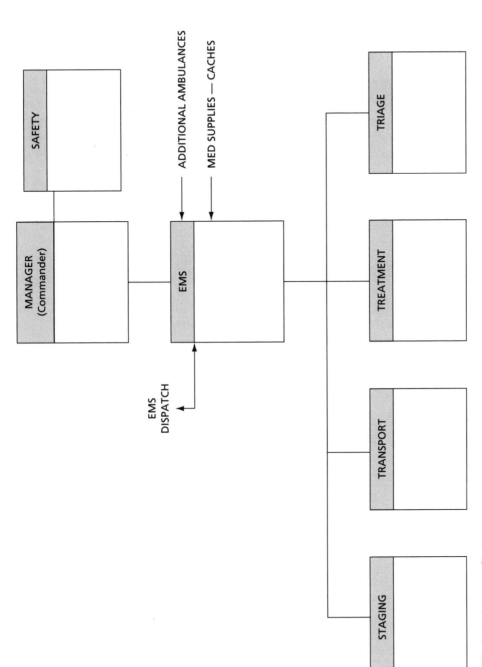

EMS Incident Mangement Chart

195

Transport Checklist

CHECKLIST: | **TRANSPORT**

RADIO CALL SIGN: "TRANSPORT"

SUPPLIES

1. VEST
2. RADIO
3. TRIAGE TAGS/RIBBONS
4. LIGHTING
5. MARKING PENS
6. GUIDESHEET
7. LZ IDENTIFICATION LIGHTING
8. SPRAYPAINT

Check	Item
	ENSURE SAFETY
	COORDINATE WITH EMS BRANCH
	TEST COMMUNICATIONS
	TRANSPORT GUIDESHEET (PATIENT DISPOSITION DATA)
	COORDINATE WITH MEDICAL COMMUNICATIONS
	ESTABLISH HELICOPTER LZ
	COORDINATE WITH TREATMENT OFFICER
	PATIENT TRACKING

INCIDENT _____   DATE _____

PATIENT DISPOSITION DATA

TIME	TAG #	SEX	NAME	HOSP	UNIT #	AGENCY	TRIAGE R-Y-G

Triage Checklist

CHECKLIST: | TRIAGE |

SUPPLIES
1. VEST
2. RADIO
3. TRIAGE TAGS/
   RIBBONS
4. LIGHTING
5. MARKING PENS

Check	Item
	ENSURE SAFETY
	COORDINATE WITH EMS BRANCH DIRECTOR
	TEST COMMUNICATIONS
	TRIAGE ALL PATIENTS
	ESTABLISH ADDITIONAL TRIAGE AREAS IF NEEDED
	DIRECT PATIENT FLOW TO TREATMENT
	MARK PATIENT FLOW WITH SCENE TAPE (IF REQUIRED)
	COORDINATE PATIENT FLOW WITH OTHER AGENCIES/ BRANCHES
	COORDINATE WITH TREATMENT

Treatment Checklist

CHECKLIST: **TREATMENT**

RADIO CALL SIGN: "TREATMENT"

SUPPLIES
1. VEST/RADIO
2. MED SUPPLIES
3. TREATMENT
   FLAGS
4. LIGHTING
5. MARKING PENS
6. SCENE RIBBON
7. PATIENT TRACKING
   DOCUMENTS

Check	Item
	ENSURE SAFETY
	COORDINATE WITH EMS BRANCH
	TEST COMMUNICATIONS
	MARK TREATMENT AREA
	COORDINATE PATIENT FLOW FROM TRIAGE
	DISASTER CACHES/RE-SUPPLY
	RED UNIT IF NEEDED
	YELLOW UNIT IF NEEDED
	GREEN UNIT IF NEEDED
	RECORD PATIENT TREATMENT
	ESTABLISH AND COORDINATE PATIENT FLOW TO TRANSPORT

Staging Checklist

CHECKLIST: STAGING

RADIO CALL SIGN: "STAGING"

SUPPLIES
1. VEST
2. RADIO
3. LIGHTING
4. UNIT TRACKING FORMS
5. MARKING PENS
6. VEHICLE KEY TAGS

Check	Item
	ENSURE SAFETY
	COORDINATE WITH EMS BRANCH
	COORDINATE WITH TRANSPORT
	TEST COMMUNICATIONS
	ESTABLISH ADEQUATE STAGING AREA
	REQUEST LAW ENFORCEMENT (IF REQUIRED)
	INVENTORY OF PERSONNEL/RESOURCES

COMMUNICATIONS CHART

AGENCY or POSITION	UNIT #	CHANNEL	FREQUENCY	CEL. PHONE	PAGER#	NOTES

INCIDENT OBJECTIVES	1. INCIDENT NAME	2. DATE PREPARED	3. TIME PREPARED

4. OPERATIONAL PERIOD (DATE/TIME)

5. GENERAL CONTROL OBJECTIVES FOR THE INCIDENT (INCLUDE ALTERNATIVES.)

6. WEATHER FORECAST FOR OPERATIONAL PERIOD

7. GENERAL/SAFETY MESSAGE

8. ATTACHMENTS (✓ IF ATTACHED)

☐ ORGANIZATION LIST (ICS 203)   ☐ MEDICAL PLAN (ICS 206)   ☐ _____

☐ DIVISION ASSIGNMENT LISTS (ICS 204)   ☐ INCIDENT MAP   ☐ _____

☐ COMMUNICATIONS PLAN (ICS 205)   ☐ TRAFFIC PLAN   ☐ _____

202 ICS 3/80	9. PREPARED BY (PLANNING SECTION CHIEF)	10. APPROVED BY (INCIDENT COMMANDER)

NFES 1326

6. SUMMARY OF CURRENT ACTIONS

ICS 201 (12/93) NFES 1325	PAGE 2	

				8. RESOURCES SUMMARY
RESOURCES ORDERED	RESOURCE IDENTIFICATION	ETA	ON SCENE	LOCATION/ASSIGNMENT
ICS 201 (12/93) NFES 1325	PAGE 4			

GLOSSARY

Agency Representative: An individual assigned to an incident by a responding or cooperating agency who is delegated complete authority to execute decisions for all dealings affecting that agency's incident participation. Representatives report to the Incident Liaison Officer.

Air Operations Branch Director: An Organization position responsible for communicating and controlling all aircraft operating in the area. Acts as an air traffic controller.

ALS (Advanced Life Support): Allowable procedures and techniques used by Paramedics and EMT-Intermediate personnel to stabilize patients who exceed basic life support procedures.

ALS Responder: Certified or licensed Paramedic or EMT/Intermediate.

Ambulance: A ground vehicle providing patient care transportation capability, specified equipment capability, and qualified personnel (EMT, EMT/I, Paramedic).

Assigned Resources: Resources checked in and assigned work tasks on an incident.

Assisting Agency: An agency directly contributing emergency medical service, fire suppression, rescue, support or service resources to another agency.

Base: Location where primary logistics functions are coordinated and administered. (Incident name or other designator should be added to the term "base" to avoid confusion.) The incident command post may be located with the base, dependent upon incident type and scope.

BLS (Basic Life Support): Basic non-invasive pre-hospital care used by Emergency Medical Technicians and the lesser trained certified First Responders to stabilize critically sick and injured patients.

BLS Responder: Certified or licensed Emergency Medical Technician, Basic or Certified First Responder.

Branch: The organizational level having functional or geographic responsibility for major segments of incident operations. The branch level is organizationally between section and group/division sectors.

Briefing: An organized face-to-face meeting between IMS managers/officers during an MCI or disaster.

C-cubed I (C³I): A military command term meaning command, control, communications, and intelligence.

Chain of Command: The flow of orders/information from the command/management level to other levels in the IMS. In effective systems, information must flow upward as well as downward.

Chemical/Biological (chem-bio) Terrorism: The use of chemical or biological weapons to create a high impact EMS incident (sometimes written as cw-bw).

Chief: Title for individuals responsible for command of functional sections: Operations, Planning, Logistics and Finance/Administration.

Clear Text/Clear Speak: The use of plain English in radio communication transmissions. No "10" codes, agency specific codes, jargon is used when using Clear Speak/Text communications.

Command: The act of directing, ordering, and/or controlling resources by virtue of explicit legal, agency, or delegated authority.

Command Cache: A kit of administrative materials and supplies necessary to operate the EMS Incident Management System; includes IMS forms, vests, checklists, and protocols.

Command Staff: The Command Staff consists of the Safety Officer, Liaison Officer, and

Public Information Officer who all report directly to the Incident Commander.

Communications Failure Protocol: A protocol that dictates agency/unit operations when there is a failure of the telephone and/or EMS radio system.

Communication Order Model: The process of briefly restating an order received to allow for verification and confirmation. This permits all involved to ensure that what was communicated actually was heard, thus ensuring that the correct action is executed.

Community Disaster Plan: A formal document that specifies who is in charge of various incidents, and what agencies/resources will be committed.

Cooperating Agency: An agency that provides indirect support or service functions, such as the American Red Cross, Salvation Army, EPA, etc.

DMAT: Disaster Medical Assistance Team, a deployable team (usually 35 people) of medical personnel and support units under the command of the Office of Emergency Preparedness, U.S. Public Health Service.

Decontamination (decon): The removal of chemical/biological/radiological contamination from responders, patients, vehicles, and equipment. Patients must be decontaminated before treatment/transport.

Delayed Patient: A patient who is stable but will require medical care; could deteriorate to the immediate category; triage color is yellow.

Disaster Cache: A store of pre-determined supplies/equipment that is immediately transported to an MCI or disaster.

Disaster-Catastrophic Incidents/Events: An MCI that overwhelms both local and regional EMS response capabilities, typically involves multiple overlapping jurisdictional boundaries, and requires significant multi-jurisdictional response and coordination.

Disaster Committee: A formal committee of response agencies, planners, support agencies, and volunteer organizations that serves as a vehicle for threat assessment, emergency response planning, disaster exercises, and post incident analysis.

Division: The organizational level having functional or geographic responsibility for major segments of incident operations.

EMS Branch: The organization level having functional responsibility for conducting emergency medical operations at a multiple casualty incident.

EMT-Basic: An individual trained in Basic Life Support according to the standards set forth by the authority having jurisdiction (local, regional, or state EMS authority).

EMT-Intermediate: An individual trained in Basic Life Support who has received additional training in Advanced Life Support according to the standards set forth by the authority having jurisdiction (local, regional, or state EMS authority).

EMT-Paramedic: An individual trained in Advanced Life Support according to the standards set forth by the authority having jurisdiction (local, regional, or state EMS authority).

Emergency Operations Center (EOC): A central disaster management center staffed by representatives from response and support agencies.

Emergency Support Functions (ESF): Support functions outlined in the Federal Response Plan. ESF's identify lead and secondary agencies and are not a management system.

Extrication Sector: The EMS IMS organizational component responsible for freeing and disentangling victims from wreckage.

Facilities Unit: Responsible for support facilities, including shelter, rehabilitation, sanitation, and auxiliary power.

Feedback: A critical element in any form of communications whereby the receiver acknowledges the receipt of information to the sender.

Firescope: Firefighting Resources of California Organized Against Potential Emergency; developed as a response to California wildfires and became the benchmark for the EMS Incident Management System.

Finance/Administration Section: The unit responsible for all costs and financial actions of the incident and administrative functions, which includes the time unit, procurement unit, compensation/claims unit, and cost unit.

General Staff: The individuals responsible for incident management, including the IM, Operations Section Chief, Logistics Section Chief, Planning Section Chief, and Administration Chief. This level is above the branch/division/group/sector level.

Ground Support Unit: The unit within the Support Branch of the Logistics Section responsible for the fueling, maintaining, and repairing of vehicles, and the transportation of personnel and supplies.

Group/Sector: The organizational level having responsibility for a specified functional assignment at an incident (triage, treatment, extrication, etc.).

Helibase: A location within the general incident area for parking, fueling, maintaining, and loading helicopters.

Helispot: A tactical location where a helicopter can take off and land.

High Impact Incident/Event: Any emergency which would require the access of mutual aid resources in order to effectively manage the incident or to maintain community 9-1-1 operations.

Hospital Alert System: A communications system between EMS personnel on-site of an MCI and a medical facility, which provides available hospital patient receiving capability and/or medical control.

Hospital Emergency Incident Command System (HEICS): A system for the management of internal/external hospital emergencies based on the IMS model.

Immediate Patient: A patient who is critical and in need of immediate care; triage color is red.

Incident Action Plan: A plan consisting of the strategic goals, tactical objectives, and support requirements for the incident. All incidents require an action plan. For simple/smaller incidents, the action plan is not usually in written form. Larger or complex responses require the action plan to be documented in writing.

Incident Command Post (ICP): The location from which command functions are executed.

Incident Management System (IMS): Originally known as the Incident Command System, IMS has evolved into a systematic management approach with a common organizational structure responsible for the management of assigned resources to effectively accomplish stated objectives pertaining to an incident.

Incident Manager (IM): The designated person with overall authority for management of the incident (varies by jurisdiction).

Incident Objectives: Statements of guidance and direction necessary for the selection of appropriate strategy(s) and the tactical direction of resources to accomplish the same. Incident objectives are based on realistic expectations of operational accomplishments when all anticipated resources have been deployed. Incident objectives must be achievable and measurable, yet flexible enough to allow for strategic and tactical realignment.

Incident Termination/Securement: The conclusion of emergency operations at the scene of an incident, usually the departure of the last resource from the incident scene.

Initial Response: The resources initially committed to an incident.

Landing Zone (LZ): A designated area to land helicopters. The LZ must be secured and controlled by a helispot manager.

Law Enforcement Incident Command System (LEICS): A law enforcement incident management system based on the IMS model.

Leader: The individual responsible for command of a task force, strike team, or unit.

Liaison: The coordination of activities between agencies operating at the incident.

Liaison Officer: The point of contact (poc) for assisting or coordinating agencies and members of the Management Staff. The Liaison Officer is a member of the Management Staff.

Logistics Section: The section responsible for providing facilities, services, and materials for the incident, which includes the communication unit, medical unit, and food unit within the Service Branch; and the supply unit, facilities unit, and ground support unit within the Support Branch.

Low Impact Incident/Event: An MCI that can be managed by local EMS resources and members without mutual aid resources from outside organizations.

Management Staff: The Incident Manager's direct support staff, consisting of the Public Information Officer, Liaison Officer, Safety Officer, and the Stress Management Officer.

Mass Casualty Incident (MCI): An incident with several patients or an unusual event associated with minimal casualties (airplane crash, terrorism, Haz Mat, etc.); incident with negative impact on hospitals, EMS, and response resources.

Mass Decontamination: The decontamination of mass numbers of patients (pediatric, adult, and geriatric) from exposure to radiation or to a chemical/biological agent.

Mechanism of Injury: A sudden and intense energy transmitted to the body that causes trauma, or exposure to a chemical or biological agent. A chem-bio mechanism of injury can be transported by a contaminated patient.

Medical Communications (EMS Com): A unit or individual that gathers on-scene patient information and transmits the information to medical control.

Medical Control: Unit responsible for monitoring and updating the patient receiving status of medical facilities in the area/region.

Medical Supply Cache: A cache consisting of standardized medical supplies and equipment stored in a predesignated location for dispatch to MCI incidents.

Medical Unit: The unit within the Service Branch of the Logistics Section responsible for providing emergency medical treatment to emergency responders. This unit does not provide treatment to civilians. Rehab is often an assigned function to the medical unit.

METTAG: A four-color system of tagging patients during the triage process. Each color is demonstrative of a differing medical priority; Red—critical, Yellow—less serious and delayed transport, Green—minor injuries (walking wounded), and Black—deceased or unsalvageable.

Minor Patient: A patient with minor injuries who requires minimal treatment; triage color is green.

Morgue: A segregated area for deceased victims that is coordinated with the Medical Examiner and/or jurisdictional law enforcement authorities; triage color for deceased victims is black.

National Interagency Incident Management System (NIIMS): An adaption of fire ICS for interagency disaster operations.

NBC: A military acronym for nuclear, biological, and chemical weapons.

Operations Section: The section responsible for all tactical operations at the incident.

Personal Protective Equipment (PPE): Equipment for the protection of EMS personnel; includes gloves, masks, goggles, gowns, and biological disposal bags (red bags).

Planning Meeting: A meeting, held as needed through the duration of the incident, to select specific strategies and tactics for incident management and for service and support planning.

Post Incident Analysis (PIA): A written review of major incidents for the purpose of implementing changes in operations, resources, logistics, and protocols, based on lessons learned.

Procurement Unit: A unit within the Finance Section responsible for financial matters involving vendors.

Public Information Officer (PIO): The person responsible for interface with the media and others requiring information direct from the incident scene. Information is only disseminated with the authorization of the Incident Manager. The PIO is a member of the Management Staff.

Pull Logistics: A process of ordering supplies by field units, via communications, as they are needed at an MCI or disaster.

Push Logistics: A process of forwarding predetermined supplies, usually as a disaster cache, to an MCI or disaster.

Real World: A phrase transmitted to all units when there is an injury or actual emergency during a disaster exercise.

Rehabilitation (Rehab): The function and location which includes medical evaluation and treatment, food and fluid replenishment, and relief from extreme environmental conditions for emergency responders, according to the circumstances of the incident.

Resource Status Unit (RESTAT): The unit within the Planning Section responsible for recording the status of, and accounting for, resources committed to the incident, and for evaluation of a.) resources currently committed to the incident, b.) the impact that additional responding units will have on an incident, and c.) anticipated resource requirements. Note: RESTAT is normally utilized at actual or escalating high-impact or long-term operations.

Safety Officer: The Management Staff member responsible for monitoring and assessing safety hazards, unsafe situations and developing measures for ensuring member safety on site.

Section: The organizational level having functional responsibility for primary segments of incident operations such as Operations, Planning, Logistics, and Finance/Administration. The section level is organizationally between Branch and Incident Manager.

Section Chief: Title referring to a member of the General Staff (Operations Section Chief, Planning Section Chief, Logistics Section Chief, and Finance/Administration Section Chief).

Sector/Group Officer: The individual responsible for supervising members who are performing a similar function or task (i.e., triage, treatment, transport, or extrication).

Security Unit: Responsible for personnel security, traffic control, and morgue security at an MCI or disaster.

Service Branch: A branch within the Logistics Section responsible for service activities at an incident. Its components include the communications unit, medical unit, and food unit.

Single Point of Contact (POC): An individual in an assisting/cooperating agency responsible for receiving and passing information and providing feedback.

Single Resource: An individual ambulance or piece of equipment used to complete a task.

Situation Status Unit (SITSTAT): The unit within the Planning Section responsible for analysis of the situation as it progresses, reporting to the Planning Section Chief. Note: SITSTAT is normally utilized at actual or escalating high-impact or long-term operations.

Span of Control: The number of subordinates supervised by a superior; ideal span varies from three to five people.

Staging: A specific status where resources are assembled in an area at or near the incident scene to await deployment or assignment.

Staging Area: The location where incident personnel and equipment are assigned on an immediately available status.

Standard Operating Procedures (SOPs): An organizational directive that establishes a standard course of action.

Standing Orders: Medical treatment policies, protocols, and procedures approved by a local, regional, or state EMS authority for use by EMS personnel without having to first make direct medical control contact for authorization.

START: Acronym for "Simple Triage And Rapid Treatment." This is an initial triage system utilized for triaging large numbers of patients at an emergency incident. This system was developed in Newport Beach, California in the early 80s.

Strategic Goals: The overall plan that will be used to control the incident. Strategic goals are broad in nature and are achieved by the completion of tactical objectives.

Strike Team: Up to five of the same kind or type of resource with common communications and an assigned leader.

Supply Unit: The unit within the Support Branch of the Logistics Section responsible for providing the personnel, equipment, and supplies to support incident operations.

Tactical Objectives: The specific operations that must be accomplished to achieve strategic goals. Tactical objectives must be specific and measurable, and are usually accomplished at the sector level.

Task Force: A group of any type or kind of resource with common communications and a leader, temporarily assembled for a specific mission (not to exceed five resources).

Technical Advisor: Any individual with specialized expertise useful to the Management/General Staff.

Technical Specialists: Personnel with special skills who are activated only when needed. Technical specialists may be needed in the areas of rescue, water resources, and training. Technical specialists report initially to the Planning Section, but may be assigned anywhere within the IMS organizational structure as needed.

Threat Assessment: An assessment of a community's vulnerability and potential for natural, technological, and terrorist risks.

Time Unit: A unit within the Finance Section responsible for record keeping of time for personnel working at an incident.

Tracking Officer: The EMS IMS organizational position, usually a sub-component of the transportation sector/group, responsible for tracking all patients removed from the scene or treated and released.

Transfer of Command: A process of transferring command responsibilities from one individual to another. Commonly a formal procedure conducted in a face-to-face interaction with an event synopsis briefing and completed by a radio transmission announcing that a certain individual is now assuming command responsibility of an incident. A similar transition occurs when a sector/group or division/branch transfers responsibilities.

Trauma Intervention Program (TIPS): A program to manage traumatic stress in emergency responders and disaster victims/families.

Transportation Sector/Group: The EMS IMS organizational component responsible for acquisition and coordination of all patient transport resources. Usually this position is responsible for coordinating the destination hospital for patients removed from the scene.

Treatment Sector/Group: The EMS IMS organizational component responsible for collecting and treating patients in a centralized location.

Triage: The act of sorting patients by the severity of their medical conditions.

Triage Sector/Group: The EMS IMS organizational component responsible for conducting triage of all patients at an MCI or high-impact incident.

Unified Command: A standard method to coordinate command of an incident when multiple agencies have either functional or geographical jurisdiction.

Unit: The organizational element having functional responsibility for a specific incident's planning, logistics, or finance activity.

Unity of Command: The concept of an individual being a supervisor at each level of the IMS, beginning at the unit level and extending upward to the Incident Manager.

INDEX